Reviews

"Dr. Lewis Rathbun has always been a masterful story teller and this is a well-told, true story of a good and caring doctor's life."

– Norma Messer, former Life After Cancer volunteer, Asheville, North Carolina.

"A life story of a physician whose dedication to his patients, outstanding medical and surgical skills and sense of humor make an inspiring narrative. Dr. Rathbun was ahead of his time in realizing the importance of the mind-body connection in the treatment of cancer patients and his Life After Cancer program is a model for compassionate care."

– H. Denniston Crews, MD, nephrologist, Asheville, North Carolina

"Readers will enjoy this good doctor's story of medicine in general and of bringing babies, in particular. In my 25 years as a health writer and editor for the *Asheville-Citizen Times* newspaper, I often turned to Dr. Rathbun for his medical expertise and wise counsel. He was generous with information, accessible and gracious. His stamp of approval was the gold standard for me. He is Asheville's Dean of Medicine."

– Nancy Marlowe, writer and editor, Asheville, North Carolina

"Dr. Rathbun is the most diversely talented individual I have ever known. Much of what I am, I owe to following as a young physician, the principles set forth in this book. Dr. Rathbun is truly a man for all seasons."

– Philip C. Davis, MD, obstetrician-gynecologist, Asheville, North Carolina

"An unaffected memoir of the pleasures and pain of being a doctor in the second half of the 20th Century. One man's goodness, skill, acceptance of all patients, and deep-seated humanism are beautifully portrayed.

"A beautiful and utterly artless portrait of a life as an obstetrician-gynecologist. Small town boyhood, Harvard Medical School, war time service in the Philippines and medical life in a Southern city—all these are captured in a gentle and delicious memoir.

"Have you ever wondered about the beauty, the perils, and the excitement of the doctor's life—especially when a father, mother and newborn are all at risk? This extraordinary book penetrates some of the great mysteries of life through the work of a distinguished obstetrician-gynecologist. The lessons are priceless."

– Daniel Federman, MD, Carl W. Walter Professor of Medicine and Medical Education, Harvard Medical School

A DOCTOR ALL MY LIFE

grateful steps
Grateful Steps
1091 Hendersonville Road
Asheville, North Carolina 28803

Rathbun, Lewis S.
A Doctor All My Life

ISBN 978-1-935130-15-4 Hard Cover

Cover design by Amy Prior
Cover portrait painting by Tucker Cooke
Cover photograph of painting by John Fletcher

Printed at BP Solutions Group, Inc.
Asheville, North Carolina

FIRST EDITION

Library of Congress Cataloging-in-Publication Data
Rathbun, Lewis, 1913-
A doctor all my life / Lewis Rathbun. -- 1st ed.
p. ; cm.
ISBN 978-1-935130-15-4 (hard cover : alk. paper)
1. Rathbun, Lewis, 1913- 2. Physicians--United States--Biography. I. Title.
[DNLM: 1. Rathbun, Lewis, 1913- 2. Physicians--United States--Personal Narratives. 3. Obstetrics--United States--Personal Narratives. WZ 100 R2338d 2009]
R154.R26 2009
610.92--dc22
[B]

2009011599

www.gratefulsteps.com

for Betty

A DOCTOR ALL MY LIFE

Lewis S. Rathbun, M.D.

Grateful Steps, Inc.
Asheville, North Carolina

ACKNOWLEDGMENTS

I wish to recognize and thank Joanna Schulman for her insistence that I write this book and for her suggestions. She gave many hours of her time, taping my dictation. I also thank Nancy Marlowe for her ideas about how to best get the book underway and for her suggestion of the book title. My daughter Laurel, an author in her own right—*Angel Pawprints; Reflections on Loving and Losing a Canine Companion* and *Angel Whiskers; Reflections on Loving and Losing a Feline Companion*—was very helpful all through this process. Much gratitude to Micki Cabaniss Eutsler and the staff at Grateful Steps for many hours, getting the material ready to go to press.

TABLE OF CONTENTS

1

GROWING UP TO BECOME A PHYSICIAN

Because he knew of my interest in becoming a doctor, Dr. Cole would take me on his Saturday house calls with him to the various farms. I would sit in his car and wait for him. We would discuss the case between stops. One day, when I was eleven or twelve years old, we were riding in the country on house calls and I was asking a barrage of questions about surgery. Dr. Cole said, "If you can find a stray cat, we'll operate on it and I'll show you how it's done." The surgery on the cat gave me a good idea of how things really work. I knew I wanted to be a surgeon.

As I look back over my life now from my present age of 95, I realize how the very early years with my family tended to shape my character, my ideas and the way I came to practice medicine.

I never agonized over what I was going to be when I grew up. I never had to "find myself" as a young man. From boyhood, I knew I wanted to be a doctor. Moreover, I wanted to be the very best physician and surgeon I could be.

Many aspects of my childhood led me toward a career in medicine. My mother was preoccupied with her health and manipulated our family with her "spells." My maiden aunt who lived with us believed she could mentally project her strength to sick people. Our progressive family doctor let me ride along on house calls and even taught me rudimentary surgery in our barn. By the time I was 12, I had fixed my hopes firmly on becoming a doctor.

I was born in 1913 in Canandaigua, New York, in the beautiful Finger Lakes area. At age two, my family moved to the farm town of Phelps in the Finger Lakes Region of Western New York. The population of Phelps was about 1600—then and now. There's an old saying that the population doesn't change because every time a baby is born, a man leaves town.

I was named Lewis Standish Rathbun. There is some distant kinship to Miles Standish. We all have heard the story of the Pilgrim founding fathers in which Miles Standish asks John Alden to propose marriage to Priscilla on his behalf. Priscilla prefers Alden and answers, "Speak for yourself, John."

This book is my effort to speak for myself about my life in medicine, then and now.

My hometown was surrounded by small farms where cabbage and grain—wheat, barley, rye—were grown. The town was a center where farmers came for supplies. My father, Alonzo Rathbun, owned and operated the town flour mill and took in the wheat. He was a merchant miller. He had his own label and sold flour to grocery stores.

The big red-brick, two-story house where we lived is now a museum that displays memorabilia from the area. Before our family lived in the house, it had been a doctor's home and there were rooms for his practice on one side. My brother Richard, who was a collector and historian, started the museum. He had returned after college to go into partnership with my father. Dick lived in the house until his death at 92.

Life was very simple. I was born into a family that was, by today's standards, very stable. My mother and father were considered fairly old when I was born. My mother was 38 and my father was 42. When I was growing up, eight of us lived in that big house—with just one bathroom. My grandparents on my father's side lived there with their unmarried daughter (my Aunt Bertha), my parents, my two brothers (who were 8 and 10 years older than I) and me. We were three generations under one roof and we got along well. I learned to value and show special concern for the elderly.

My grandmother and grandfather celebrated their 50th wedding anniversary in that house. My mother and father lived together for 62 years, both my brothers observed their 50th anniversaries and I have since celebrated mine and am coming up on my 70th.

Family life was peaceful. My grandmother and grandfather did not interfere with the family dynamics. They almost never made suggestions as to how to bring up the boys or what mother and father should do. I think that they must have decided as long as they had to live with us, they would make a conscious effort not to. That certainly made it more pleasant than some families I've seen where several generations live together. My grandmother and grandfather became very feeble, and I remember very well having to help them around the house, getting them up and down the stairs. I think this instilled in me a feeling that I ought to be helping people.

My father didn't enter into a lot of family things. He would come home at night and read *The Saturday*

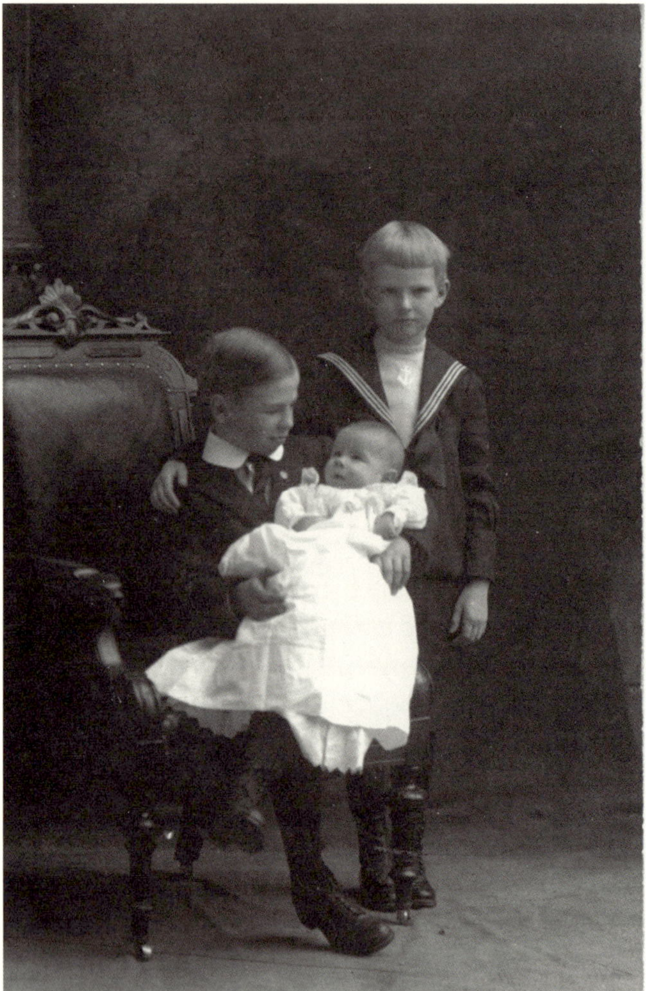

Baby Lewis Standish Rathbun
with brothers (L to R)
Herbert Douglas and Richard Lee

Evening Post from beginning to end, and my mother would talk on and on and then say, "Why, you haven't heard a thing I've said." I never remembered any violent quarrels between them. This has influenced me through the years. I have always thought it better to get along with people than to quarrel with them, even if it means giving up a few things along the way.

In my early childhood, there were no cars in the town. It is interesting to look back at a picture of life then. We walked everywhere. It was just a couple of blocks to the stores and businesses—Mom 'n Pop things—along Main Street.

At noon, we had an hour off from school. We walked home for lunch and then walked back. After school, the farm kids worked on their farms. There was only one fat kid in the whole school.

People traveled mainly by trains. A branch of the New York Central Railroad ran through town, the rails stretching on to Geneva and Rochester. Women from Phelps routinely rode the nine miles to Geneva on the train, did their shopping and caught the train home four hours later.

I have fond memories of my father's first car. My maternal grandfather lived in Oneida, 90 miles away. He was a very successful businessman—a grocery wholesaler and bank president. In about 1919, he bought my father a car. Father went to Oneida on the train to get the car. He had never driven a car before so my grandfather drove around the block with him and then my father headed home for Phelps.

Normally, one didn't drive a car any great distance in those days. In winter, we didn't drive at all. There were no snow plows. Therefore, roads—largely unpaved outside of town—were essentially impassable from mid-November on into April. The car was jacked up on blocks in the garage or barn in November and stayed there until spring. The farmers put sled runners on the wagons and used the wagons for getting around. Parents bringing children into town for school had horse-drawn sleighs called cutters. Rides in these cutters were an adventure.

My mother was something of a hypochondriac and regularly had what we called her "weak spells."

"I'm just all used up," Mother would say, announcing one of her spells. She would then take to her bed for a few hours or a few days.

The family accepted these episodes. My Aunt Bertha, who was a spiritual woman, tried to help my mother. My aunt believed she could help sick or weak people by projecting her own health and strength onto them. Aunt Bertha had helped others in this way . . . or thought she did. She was a very strong individual and she had a deep faith which did not necessarily follow the church rules. She felt that there was something to extrasensory perception and that she had a gift for it. I saw several indications through time that she seemed able to sense what was going on and communicate things. That impressed me. If somebody outside the family was desperately ill, she would retire into her room and relax and concentrate on filling them with strength. There did seem to be something to what she was doing, and it interested me tremendously as I was growing up. Mother seemed to think Aunt Bertha helped her, but it never lasted.

I had not heard the word psychosomatic at the time, but I saw evidence of it in my own family. My mother's "weak spells" went back to her adolescence. At 12 or 14, she fainted for some unknown reason and was kept out of school for a few days. She ended up staying out of school a whole semester with a minor or imaginary illness.

Our family was resigned to mother's spells. There was always the talk, "Well, we can't do this because mother isn't well." I saw very early in the game that she was using illness to get her way, and she was very efficient at it. On occasion I confronted her with this. The first hormone shots, which I learned later through authoritative sources were not very effective, came out sometime around 1928. Armed with a new intervention, her doctor, who I'm sure was at his wit's end trying to do something for Mother, said to her, "Let's try this."

She would walk up to his office about a block away to get the shots. I noticed that when she was walking up there, she was walking slowly, obviously weak, depressed and not feeling well. She would get the shot and then come almost prancing down the street, swinging her arms and remarking how the shots picked her up and how she felt so much better. I was only 14 or 15 at the time. I said, "You know, nothing he has given you can work so fast!" She was very upset with me about that. In fact, I used to be somewhat unpopular with the whole family for suggesting that the shots weren't doing what they thought they were. I know now that it was the "placebo effect" that was working. I also know now that my mother's spells were probably not deliberate manipulation but her mechanism of coping, defending herself against whatever she feared.

So at an early age, I recognized the mind's effect on the body. Early in my adolescence I began to wonder about the role of emotions in diseases. As I went to medical school and began to practice, the interest became more and more intense, and as research began to come out on it, I was very interested. This eventually led to my founding a group called Life After Cancer/Pathways in which I participated for twenty-two years and acquired a great deal of knowledge about how the emotions can affect the immune system and the disease of cancer.

In the course of Mother's illness, the two doctors in town became well known to me. One was old and didn't have much of a practice. The other, Dr. Kenneth Cole, was just out of his medical training. He was at the house a lot to see both my mother with her difficulties with psychosomatic type illnesses and my grandmother with various illnesses of old age. He became a mentor—but I didn't think of it that way then. At an early age I began to think about diseases and what caused them and asked him many questions about them.

When he was taking my mother's pulse or my grandmother's blood pressure, he'd show me how to do it. This was about 1925, and the country roads were pretty good in the summer by then.

Dr. Cole was a short, trim, good-looking man with a mustache. He had a friendly, unhurried manner. I remember one day we met the rural-route mailman on his rounds. Dr. Cole teased the mailman, saying, "I just delivered Mrs. So-and-So. I looked the baby over pretty closely for a postage stamp!"

There were no hospitals in our town but there were two very near—about 15 miles away—that he worked in. In those days, general practitioners in small towns did their own surgery. This fascinated me.

Because he knew of my interest in becoming a doctor, Dr. Cole would take me on his Saturday house calls with him to the various farms. I would sit in his car and wait for him. We would discuss the case between stops. One day, when I was about eleven or twelve years old, we were riding in the country on house calls and I was asking a barrage of questions about surgery. Dr. Cole said, "If you can find a stray cat, we'll operate on it and I'll show you how it's done."

I soon located a barn cat that nobody wanted. Dr. Cole and I set up an operating room in the barn where my father parked his car. We anesthetized the cat with chloroform and took out the appendix and the gallbladder and then opened the chest and watched the heart work. We put the cat to sleep with an overdose of chloroform. Just then, my dad drove in and was amazed to see the barn had been turned into an operating theater.

The surgery on the cat gave me a good idea of how things really work. I knew I wanted to be a surgeon.

Later on, when I was in my second year in medical school, Dr. Cole arranged for me to deliver a baby. I was riding with him on house calls when I was home from medical school on vacation. A girl I had gone to high school with was in the throes of labor. Dr. Cole checked her and said to me that she was not going to deliver for some time. He told me he would leave me and his bag there to reassure her as he slipped out to the next patient on his rounds.

The baby came right away. I delivered it and all went very well. I knew Dr. Cole had planned it that way.

That day I would not have believed that, many years later, I would assist Dr. Cole in surgery in Coral Gables, Florida, where he had moved after he left Phelps. That would happen when I was a full-fledged doctor attending a medical convention in nearby Miami Beach.

My boyhood in Phelps included lots of tramping around the countryside with other boys and enjoying nature. We did some trapping of muskrats and skunks. In those days, we could sell skunk pelts. I guess that skinning the muskrats and skunks was really my first surgery experience. As I look back on it, I regret trapping the animals. I didn't understand at the time how they suffered in the traps. Muskrats were famous for chewing through their legs. I'd find a trap with a foot in it. If I had just thought about it, I could have changed. It was a whole bunch of boys who went trapping together. It was just something boys did.

I often went along on hunting trips, but I never carried a gun. I just enjoyed being out in the fields and seeing the pheasants and other living creatures. I later came to observe wildlife through the lens of the camera. Nature became my source of subjects for many of the watercolor paintings I did in midlife.

Father was busy with his flour milling business and didn't pay much attention to his children. He never played sports, such as "catch," with me. When I got into high school he would drive me to the basketball games. I always had an interest in sports but never was very good at them and never made any of the teams. But my lanky build and the muscles I developed in my legs as a country boy worked to my advantage. In college I got a letter in track—my only accomplishment in the area of sports.

Phelps was quite a friendly place. People helped each other when they were in trouble. In my childhood, Phelps had several grocery stores. Main Street was about a mile and a half long and was divided into the east and west end. The east end had the big houses, and the west end had the smaller houses of the working people. There was no industry there as I grew up other than small canning factories, mostly producing sauerkraut. A lot of cabbage was grown in the area. At harvest time, horse-drawn wagons filled with heads of cabbage were backed up all the way to our house. We lived at the east end of Main Street and a big sauerkraut factory was at the other end. As little boys, we would go out and ask one of the drivers for a cabbage and they would always throw us one.

The only school in Phelps would never pass muster now. I remember it as a three-story, square brick building with a wooden stairwell up the center. In the basement under the stairwell was a furnace. It is amazing that the place never burned down. It wasn't the simplest school in the area at the time, however. There were one-room school houses out in the countryside to which some of the farm kids went.

I was a pretty fair student. I got good marks. The courses I liked in high school—biology, chemistry and physics—were what I needed for medical school. I liked English and history well enough and did well in math, but I was not much good in foreign languages.

I was involved in various plays in school. Although I was not typically the leading man, I was one of the few who weren't scared to be on stage, so I got good parts. Each graduating class had a senior play. The entire town attended. In one play I had to put my arm around a girl. I was so self-conscious about it that I didn't act the part very well. In another play a fellow across the room was supposed to toss me a can of tobacco. I missed it and it went sailing across my shoe. I had been in a seated position and instead of getting up and getting it, I just sat there and went on with the script. I was questioned a lot about that later.

For a while Phelps had a movie theater. Although movies were pretty sour in those days, I was so impressed. Heroes would be out on wings of airplanes and would reach and catch the heroine. I thought it was well worth my ten cents. My mother thought it was awful. The minister's daughter played the piano for the theater, causing some consternation in the Presbyterian Church.

COLLEGE

After I graduated from high school in Phelps, I enrolled in Hamilton College in Clinton, New York. My two brothers had gone there before me, and I never considered any place else. It was a small college in those days—about 450 students, all men. Now it has about 1500 students and is coed.

A good deal of the college education was done in the fraternity house. It was a major growth experience to come from a small town with a fairly small group of friends and a small high school and to start living in a fraternity house with thirty boys from all different walks of life. I learned to get along with men of different backgrounds with different ideas and different values. I learned not to be judgmental about them and came to realize that such differences were part of living out there in the world.

A few of the fraternity brothers were from affluent homes. Most were upper middle class. All of us, however, were affected by the Depression which was at its height in 1931. There was a great deal of learning to be done about how to live with different people and get along with them. Some of the rules of the fraternity were quite strict and seemed positive to me at the time, although I don't think they are followed nowadays. For instance, we had to wear a coat and tie at dinner each night. Some of the boys had only one or two jackets or suits.

We were very careful about speaking correct English in the fraternity house. This was part of working toward the goal of learning to live in correct society. If we used the wrong verb or tense, someone would yell at us. It was a good education to watch and see why some boys were popular and some were not and then to distill out of that, modifications in my own actions and my own way of living.

Hamilton was a small college out in the country, and there were no girls' colleges anywhere near it. It was possible to go to Utica and back—a nine-mile trolley ride away—for twenty cents. Saturday afternoon and evening a movie cost fifteen cents, and maybe we could get a sparse dinner for thirty-five cents. That was about all most of our budgets would handle in the height of the Depression. There was almost no drinking around the fraternity house. This was during Prohibition. After the college games and other group activities, nobody thought of having any liquor around. There was a speakeasy fairly near the college, which a few of the boys frequented, but it was expensive and most of us didn't have the money or the desire to drink.

The Depression molded me; I found that I had to work hard for whatever I could get. I was very willing to work at extra jobs—washing dishes in the fraternity, working on farms in the summer. I found in those days that hard work paid off. It formed a basis for a work ethic that I carried through my life.

We went to sports events—football, basketball, track, baseball and tennis. The college had a good sports program, and the particular activities they pushed could be useful for a lifetime. For example, there was a rule that in order to graduate one had to do a certain number of hours of tennis, golf and skiing.

In fall and spring, we had a house party, which consisted of girls coming in from various places on Friday. Each boy invited a date. We cleared out the fraternity houses so they could be used as the girls' sleeping quarters. The boys doubled up in the dorms.

Each fraternity house had a band. The dances were all formal; we wore tuxes and tails. In spite of the Depression, tails were quite popular. I had a hand-me-down tux from my brother that didn't fit very well. I desperately hoped someday to own a set of tails. At about the end of my second year in college, the only really wealthy man in Phelps—who lived two doors from us and was friendly with my family—heard how badly I wanted some formal attire and gave me fifty dollars, which at that time was just the right amount to buy a set of tails. That was one of the big events in my life—going into Utica, getting a set of tails and being outfitted for the house party that spring.

The college curriculum was designed to give a broad-based education. In the first two years, there was a required variety of courses, including Romance languages, English, math and sciences. After that, the student could specialize in whatever he wanted. I enjoyed most of my studies, especially the science ones—chemistry, math and biology. Just as in high school, I did not enjoy the languages. I never was very good at them. It took a lot of work to get through them. In contrast, I immensely enjoyed the philosophy courses. In fact, I took enough of the philosophy courses to have a major in it. However, the two majors that were required for my premed work were biology and chemistry.

Looking back, I think that one of the things I liked about the philosophy courses was the chance to do some original thinking—questioning why things happened and learning how to figure things out for myself. In most of the courses I had taken up until that time, the student simply learned things that were in the book. The emphasis was on chemical formulas in chemistry and how the stomach worked in physiology. It was all about committing facts to memory. In philosophy, I could read the words of the great thinkers handed down through the ages and then distill the information and make up my own philosophy of life from that.

I enjoyed physics both in high school and in college, although it was a science that many people seemed to find difficult. I thought it was extremely interesting to find out why and how things worked and how the various laws of the universe were applied to make them happen.

I guess biology was my main love in college. Of course, it helped that it was connected with my interest in medicine. We had an outstanding professor, a fairly young man who was doing research on the endocrine system. He took an interest in those of us who demonstrated that we wanted to learn all we could. We took some of the advanced classes, which later helped us in medical school, such as embryology and bacteriology, classes one wouldn't ordinarily get in college. I worked with him on some of his research and got to know him very well. I attributed to his excellent teaching the high marks I received in biology.

Harvard was known across the country at that time, as it still is, as one of the top medical schools in the country and probably in the world. When it came time for those of us in premed to apply to medical school, the biology professor was well positioned to help us get into Harvard. There were several Hamilton students who had been accepted there before and who had done very well.

There were more applicants for the good schools than they could take. Therefore, most of us applied to several schools, but Harvard was typically the first choice. I remember applying at Harvard, Yale, Columbia, Vanderbilt and University of Rochester. The medical schools picked up their chosen applicants at different times during the year. It was like a game of roulette. Some of the medical schools that were less desirable selected early in the hope that the students would be afraid to wait for some of the better ones. I decided to wait until I heard from Harvard. Fortunately, about the first of February, 1935, I heard from my top choice early. It was a very happy time. This had been one of my desires for a long time and now was almost within my grasp. I felt that there I would get the best possible education to become the best doctor that I could be.

During my four years at Hamilton, I developed a feeling of great pride for my college that has lasted. I felt the school was going all out to get me the best education at the cheapest price. I had scholarships and worked a variety of jobs throughout my time there to help cover expenses. I still feel a little perturbed when I ask some of my classmates, on behalf of the college, to contribute to the annual fund. I get answers that indicate that they don't feel they owe the college anything. But I do. After more than 65 years, I still feel a deep loyalty to Hamilton.

In the summer after graduating from college, I worked near home in Clifton Springs at a hospital laboratory. I worked for no pay because the hospital was in bad financial straits due to the Depression. I learned to cut sections from the medical specimens and prepare them for the pathologist. The pathologist—a skilled Hopkins-trained physician and an excellent teacher—in turn, would tell me about the specimens and the diseases, preparing my way for the medical training ahead of me. He began letting me do autopsies under his supervision. So when I began my pathology rotation at medical school, I had a head start.

2

MEDICAL EDUCATION

One of the highlights of the third year came in early fall when I was assigned to the obstetrical service out in the district. The Boston Lying-In Hospital had an arrangement for delivering babies in the tenements. The medical school owned two houses. One was behind Mass General in East Boston. The other was in South Boston. The students lived there two weeks, having first been prepared at the Boston Lying-In Hospital where we had observed deliveries. My first delivery occurred on my birthday. As I left the tenement area just as dawn was breaking, I had the feeling that by delivering a baby on my birthday, I had paid back something to the country . . . or the universe. I can still remember that feeling of accomplishment that day.

MEDICAL SCHOOL

The day finally came when I started for Boston and Harvard Medical School. I went on the train alone that

September day in 1935. When I got out to the medical school by taxi and went on to the dorm, I remember very clearly the exhilaration and happiness I felt as I carried my suitcase up the steps and into Vanderbilt Hall, the dormitory for medical students. Here I was, finally, at what I consider to be one of the best medical schools in the world and about to start something I had looked forward to for so long—my medical education and the chance to become a full-fledged M.D. I had a great feeling of elation that I was finally here and my dream was about to come true. I was determined to do well and be the best doctor I could be.

First Year

When classes started, the most concentrated work of my life began—studying every night except Saturday night and working hard through the day in various laboratories and lectures. However, as hard as it was and as unaccustomed as almost all of us were to this concentrated work that we had not had in college, I was happy to do it and never thought that I was being put upon. It was all part of accomplishing what I had started out to do. The professors—for the most part—were excellent and renowned people whom I could look up to and feel privileged to work under.

My classmates and I came in as freshmen in the same year that Dr. James Bryan Conant, the renowned chemist, was installed as president of Harvard University. What exactly led to his selection for the position, I'm not sure. Not long after we arrived, we were called together and Dr. Conant addressed us. This wasn't the head of the medical school; this was the head of the university. I remember being surprised at one thing he said. He did not think that a broad education was necessary to go into medical school. He personally believed that people who knew they wanted to be doctors should just spend two years in college and take nothing but the courses necessary to prepare them for medical school.

Having just graduated from Hamilton, where we had to have a broad education no matter what we were going to do, I felt—despite respect for this great man and educator—that he was wrong in this. He may have been a great chemist and a great head of the university, but he was wrong in not pushing for people to have a very broad educational base for living. I took a third major in philosophy just because I was interested. I didn't need it. I only needed chemistry and biology. I still feel that the education I got at Hamilton—including English and history and political science and various other courses that had nothing to do with getting into medical school—has stood me in very good stead throughout my life, broadening me to the point that I can appreciate life fully and therefore, be a better physician.

Our classes started with Anatomy—both Microscopic and Gross. The laboratory area consisted of very large rooms, each with four dissecting tables. On each table was a cadaver. We were assigned in groups of four to a cadaver. Each team of four was together all the way through the first term.

The room smelled of formaldehyde. We wore smocks. We were at first hesitant to begin dissection, but it soon became very interesting to see the various organs and to learn the paths of the nerves and blood vessels. Almost immediately, I realized that we had to study a lot differently from the way we did in college. I got into the habit, as did most of the other students, of having dinner and then going up into the common room for a few minutes and then about 7:30, sitting down at my desk and studying through to 11 or 11:30 each night, almost without interruption. There was no visiting back and forth between the rooms or anything like that. It was just pure study and memorization, but something I found to be pleasant, not drudgery.

For the first two years, we had lectures and laboratory work all day Monday through Friday and half a day on Saturday. Nowadays, the Saturdays have been cut out. On Saturdays, in order to give us a little taste of clinical activities, we met at the amphitheater of Peter Bent Brigham Hospital. One of the professors of either Surgery or Medicine would present a case to us. An actual patient would be wheeled into the classroom. The professor would talk about the disease and how it was diagnosed and treated. We weren't expected to take notes or be examined on this at all; it was simply to give us an exposure to patients. These sessions were a highlight of our week because having nothing but cadavers and laboratory work to do seemed quite removed from actual medicine. This brought us into contact with "real" medicine and was as much a morale builder as anything we did.

Saturday afternoons, most of us took off. I got a job as an usher at Harvard Stadium when the football team was playing at home, so I was able to see the games for nothing. Saturday night, most of us would go downtown to a movie. The Depression was still on and money was extremely scarce, not just for me, but for most of us. We were careful how we spent it. Movies were cheap at twenty-five cents.

Sunday morning, I frequently went to church and then had dinner at the dorm. In the afternoon, we stayed in the common room and talked until about three o'clock and then most of us disappeared to study. This is completely different from the way I understand students live now.

There were no female professors or classmates. In fact they didn't accept applications. "Nothing against women," the Dean of Admissions said. "It is a matter of simple statistics. The average female only practices half the time that the men do. We have 3000 to 4000 applications for 125 places, so we do not want to waste the education provided for half the returns." Now the majority of students are women.

There were no blacks among the medical students, either. "Because they do not have the educational background to get in," the Dean explained. We had exposure to only one black professor. Professor Hilton developed a test for syphilis that was better than the Wasserman, although more complicated to perform. He came as a visiting lecturer to talk to us about it. Afro-Americans were admitted later because of government pressure so the school could get grants. When Harvard began admitting black students, they were initially asked to arrive mid-June and work all summer to "get up to the white boys." Now there are lots of black men and women in Harvard Medical School, and they don't need to come early.

Second Year

The second year we began to learn actual medicine. I vividly remember one lecture. Sulfanilamide, the first of the antibiotics, had been discovered about six months earlier. We had a lecture from one of the well known surgeons in Boston about streptococcus infections and how sulfa drugs were showing progress. At the end of his lecture on streptococcus he said, "I suppose I should mention the drug that is in all the newspapers, but I wouldn't worry about it. I have seen these things come and go over the years. Somebody thinks they have something great, and then in six months you never hear of it again because it doesn't work. In fact," he said, "I just bet another physician $100 that in six months you would not hear anything more about sulfanilamide." I've often wondered whether he paid the debt or not.

We worked on the wards, large patient units with as many as 40 beds, as part of our Physical Diagnosis course, an interesting first-exposure to patients in the hospital setting. Patients stayed longer than they do today. For example, cardiac patients might be there three to four weeks. We had a great deal of cases of rheumatic fever, which could cause major heart murmurs and serious heart-chamber enlargements. We learned to listen to diagnose these disorders. Many of these patients must have become pretty tired of having us come in and auscultate their hearts. They already had their regular intern, assistant resident, senior resident and visiting man listening to them and making records on them and now, medical students fumbling around with them. It is surprising how accommodating they were despite what may not have been a happy experience, especially if they were quite sick.

The instructor would pick out a patient with an interesting clinical finding and would teach at the bedside. This is where we learned physical diagnosis, divided into groups of eight. We were dependent on clinical skills, such as percussion and listening for transmission of spoken sound to the auscultated lung fields. This is a lost art now; imaging resolves diagnostic dilemmas and replaces much of those skills.

We would ask the patients to say, "ninety-nine, ninety-nine, ninety-nine," and would simultaneously listen to their lungs with a stethoscope, distinguishing between open air space and consolidation by the sound we heard. One man, located halfway down the room, had been in the ward for a long time. He had been examined time after time by medical students. As we entered one day, he called out to the fellow in the bed across from him, "Hey, Charlie, wake up! Ninety-nine, ninety-nine, ninety-nine!"

Our teachers for clinical medicine were called "visiting men." They were assigned in rotation—to supervise our care and educate us in the process. There were no "visiting women" during my training. The visiting faculty were typically physicians in private practice outside the hospital or academicians doing research at the university. They were under the professors and associate professors as far as lines of administration and authority at the medical school.

We were at the beginning steps of learning a vast amount of material that forms the basis for clinical medicine—learning that would continue throughout our lives as physicians. One day, our Physical Diagnosis instructor took us off the floor where we were working with cardiac patients and took us up to another level, where he presented us with a woman about 35 years of age who had a variety of symptoms. He asked us each to examine her. She had a very large mass in her abdomen, and of course, we all found the mass. Then when we started talking about what it could be, we all had varying diagnoses. Not one of us picked up on the fact that it was a pregnancy! The instructor pointed out to us that we can get so fixated on one diagnosis while examining a patient that we skip some of the obvious findings that are there. Lessons like these made a lasting impression, even if the context was somewhat to our chagrin.

Third Year

One of the highlights of the third year came in early fall when I was assigned to the obstetrical service out in the district. The Boston Lying-In Hospital had an arrangement for delivering babies in the tenements. The medical school owned two houses. One was behind Mass General in East Boston, an area that was all slums then. Now that is all gone, replaced by businesses and very expensive condominiums. The district it served extended from near old North Church over to Charles River. The other was in South Boston. Each had a housekeeper and two students. The students lived there two weeks, having first been prepared at the Boston Lying-In Hospital where we had observed deliveries and perhaps would have the opportunity to actually do one. We ran prenatal clinics in the area to be sure the mothers-to-be were healthy. In fact, pregnant women were not eligible for the home-delivery program if they had not attended the prenatal clinic. The assistant resident stayed there a month at a time and ran a prenatal clinic. There were 29,000 deliveries without a maternal death attributable to prenatal clinics.

In the East unit, at the McLean house on McLean Street, the unmarried woman who was housekeeper was still there when I returned as a resident. She had been there for years and often answered the phone, "No hurry" or "Better get out here right away." She knew the patients well.

Patients called when they were in active labor, and we went out, took care of them and delivered their babies. This was the first time we had any real experience with responsibility for patients of our own. It was both thrilling and terrifying.

Most of us delivered from ten to twelve babies in the course of two weeks. We had a public health nurse who accompanied us. I was amazed at the deference shown us by the people in the tenements. The husbands were usually there, and sometimes three or four other children standing behind us as we delivered the babies. We stayed through the whole labor, checking the patient's progress. The laboring women had no anesthesia.

If we sensed some trouble, we would call the resident who was the next in the line of hierarchy over us at the hospital. If he couldn't handle the situation, he would call one of the younger visiting men who would sometimes come out and see what was going on. Of course, if it got into serious trouble, we called an ambulance and sent the patient directly to the Lying-In.

I felt fortunate that all of my deliveries went smoothly. I enjoyed getting to know the people. We had to go back and see them after the births, of course. We made house calls every day for about ten days. We did the women a favor by taking care of them and delivering them, but they also did us a favor by subtly showing us how to handle patients. If it was a third or fourth or fifth baby, the fathers knew more about it than we did. If we exercised restraint and humility, we could learn from them.

We sometimes got a little bit intimidated by some of the families. I remember one father who said, "We drink to the baby? Huh, Doc?"

I didn't want to be impolite so I said, "Yes, we'll drink to the baby." He got out a bottle of clear liquid. He poured himself half a glass and poured me a shot glass full and gave it to me. He promptly drank his down and I thought, "Well, this can't be so bad." So, I tossed the contents of the shot glass back into my mouth and drank with one swallow. It was about ten minutes before I could breathe again! The clear liquid was anisette—a very potent liqueur.

As long as we had our black bags, which identified us not only as physicians, but probably out on a delivery call, we were perfectly safe walking around in the streets or up in the tenement houses—day or night. We never had any fear. I suspect that nowadays, walking around in an area like that in one of the big cities, one would probably be lucky if he were not killed for the possibility of having drugs in the bag. We experienced none of that. Not only were we safe, but people were repeatedly helpful when we needed to locate a patient or confirm an address.

My first delivery occurred on my birthday. As I left the tenement area just as dawn was breaking, I had the feeling that by delivering a baby on my 22nd birthday, I had paid back something to the country . . . or the universe. I can still remember that feeling of accomplishment that day.

Boston had three big teaching hospitals when I was there: Peter Bent Brigham, Boston Lying-In and The Free Hospital for Women. Now, Brigham and Women's Hospital combines all three. The Free Hospital for Women was just for gynecology problems. Ward patients who had received care in the outpatient department could be scheduled there. It had no emergency room. It had been free since its conception in the 1800s. Boston Lying-In was entirely for obstetrics. Approximately 5500 deliveries were performed a year in the mid-1930s. The other hospitals were Massachusetts General, referred to as "Mass General," and Boston City Hospital. It is now the medical school, research buildings and high school. It was noted for care of cancer patients.

The third year of medical school brought our first experience in the operating room. We started with a series of instructions on how to scrub our hands, how to move around in the operating room without touching things and contaminating them and how to get into our gowns and gloves without touching the outside surfaces. Only then were we allowed to participate in the operation. Granted, we were pretty far down the table from the actual procedure, since there was a chief surgeon, a resident and a scrub nurse, all of whom really knew what was going on. But we did get to hold retractors and listen to the comments of the surgeon. We were intent on picking up any words of instruction.

I felt privileged to be on the operating team of two of the best-known surgeons in the medical school, and indeed, in the country—Dr. Elliot Carr Cutler, full professor of surgery, and Dr. Holmans, who had written a widely-used textbook of surgery. They were good instructors while they were operating. This increased my interest in surgery and also took me back to my first operation—on the cat.

While on the Surgery service, we gained experience on the wards—both in preoperative diagnosis and postoperative care. Wards were hospital patient units consisting of large rooms with numerous beds separated by curtains. We were slowly getting closer and closer to being a doctor, able to take care of patients for whom we were personally responsible.

During the work in the third year on the Medicine Service, we were assigned patients on the medical wards. We did the histories and physicals and—along with the other house staff—made physical diagnoses. We didn't write any orders on the patients but studied what was ordered on them and made rounds with the visiting man on the whole ward so that we knew what was going on with all the patients.

We had our first experience with people who had fatal diseases, such as severe untreatable heart trouble and various other diseases which were fatal then but are not fatal now. We learned what patients went through as they knew they were dying.

The work on the wards while on both Medicine and Surgery services was interspersed with lectures by professors and specialists in certain diseases. We were gradually becoming knowledgeable about the science of medicine as it was at that time. Most of us began to decide in which branch of medicine we would eventually specialize. I had enjoyed both surgery and obstetrics and felt that I would be happy in Ob-gyn, which encompassed both of those aspects of medicine. For one thing, obstetrical patients were young and by-and-large happy people. I had decided that I would not like orthopedics, where, in those days, the clinician would put somebody in a cast and have to see them for what seemed to be months on end. This did not appeal to me at all.

So, I set my course to specialize in obstetrics and gynecology.

Fourth Year

The last year was probably the easiest of the four. We had learned to study and get around the hospital. There wasn't as much memorization work as there was patient observation and listening to lectures. In the fourth year, we worked in both the surgical and medical outpatient departments at the hospitals and saw an entirely different type of patient from those we had seen working on the wards in the third year. I remember being at Boston City Hospital in the surgical outpatient unit during the winter. Boston had a rule that if there was snow to be cleared in the streets, the men on welfare were pressed into service to help with the snow shoveling. Equipment in those days was not as efficient as it is now. Snow removal was hard labor. One can be sure that on any morning when heavy snow had to be cleared, the surgical outpatient area at the Boston City Hospital would be filled with men on welfare complaining about all sorts of back problems so that they could get a slip saying that they were unable to shovel snow on that day. That added to our knowledge of human nature and what we might expect in our practices.

There was an attending surgeon named Dan. We didn't like him because he would perform the surgery on the residents' cases when he was on duty at Boston Lying-In—we would only assist. When I was chief resident, he and I did not do well together at all. I recall a woman with membranes ruptured for one to two days who needed a "Waters section"—delivery of her baby from the abdominal route using a technique designed for the setting of a serious infection risk for the mother in a time when no antibiotics were available. It would be a difficult operation. All the residents were anxious to do as many as possible. We needed to use care pulling infected tissues out of the abdomen. Dan was the visiting man on service, and I knew if he did the surgery, I would only be watching. So I called our department chairman, Dr. Frederick C. Irving. "There is a case up here you might want to see."

Dr. Irving, known by all trainees as "The Professor," came to the unit and asked me to schedule the procedure with him. (Sometimes enhancing my education was simply a matter of clever engineering.) We did an extraperitoneal cesarean section, developed at a New Jersey Hospital. In that operation, the uterus was isolated from the abdominal contents so that the mother's organs weren't exposed to the infectious organisms in the uterine cavity.

We had some time in our fourth year to take some elective courses. We could take whatever appealed to us. We could learn more about certain diseases or we could even do some research. I elected to take a month's course in cancer pathology. Already at that early time, I was very interested in cancer and wanted to learn as much about it as I could. I was very lucky to be chosen for a course under Dr. Shields Warren who was one of the top cancer pathologists in the country. He was later chosen to head the pathology studies involved in the Manhattan Project when the first nuclear weapons were developed during World War II.

The cancer course was extremely interesting to me. There were only three or four students, so Dr. Warren spent a great deal of time with us individually—talking to us and reviewing slides. At that time we thought we knew a great deal about cancer, but now I realize we had only scratched the surface.

The middle part of the fourth year was largely consumed with the matter of getting an internship. The year or two of work in hospitals that was called an internship was designed to prepare the graduate physician with a broad hands-on training in preparation for the more specialized residency years or for general practice. Now the internship has largely disappeared, that goal having been met in the fourth year of medical school and the first year of residency.

In the late '30s, the process was not as well structured as it is today. The hospitals with positions open chose interns at various times. The hospitals did not pick their interns all at once as they do now. It was harrowing for the students. Some of the better positions became available after some of the less desirable ones. If a student waited for the premier appointments, there was a significant chance of not getting anything very good at all in the area of medicine that he really wanted. At that time, the obstetrics-gynecology residencies to which I aspired at the Boston Lying-In and the Free Hospital for Women insisted on a two-year surgical internship before accepting applications. The professors wanted the trainee to already be able to operate without any problem before learning their techniques.

I applied for what I felt was a very excellent internship at Strong Memorial Hospital at the University of Rochester in Rochester, New York. It was a two-year surgical internship that had a little obstetrics and gynecology in it. This would satisfy the requirements of the Boston Lying-In and the Free Hospital. I also applied for the surgical internships at Yale and at Vanderbilt.

As part of my application to Yale, I asked Dr. John Homans if he would write a letter of recommendation, since that was a school at which he had been Professor of Surgery. When I entered his office, he had his feet on the desk. "What do you want? I don't know you."

"I was on your service three months last summer. Perhaps you could ask the residents about me. It would mean a great deal . . . for my application to Yale since you were a professor there."

He glared, "All right. I'll write your recommendation—write a god-damn good one! Goodbye."

Dr. Homans was notorious on the surgical service. At Brigham, there was a long corridor with six operating rooms on each side of the hall, and the doctors' dressing room was at the far end. Dr. Homans would come out of the doctors' dressing room half-dressed, always in a rush to go back to the hospital. He would still be tucking in his shirt tail and buttoning his pants. By the time he reached the hospital doors, he would be fairly well put together.

One day, the Operating Room Supervisor had seen about enough. She said, "Dr. Homans, I wish you'd dress before you leave the dressing room. I have a lot of student nurses. You scare them when you come out still buttoning up your pants."

He never broke his stride. "Tell your student nurses the time to be scared of a man is when he is *unbuttoning* his pants, not when he is buttoning them!"

I didn't apply in Boston for an internship. The Boston openings were very sought-after. The selections did not occur until very late in the year and I was afraid if I didn't get one, I would be left out and have to take a very inferior internship.

I waited. Fortunately, I heard fairly soon that I had gotten into the University of Rochester—my first choice—so that problem was settled during the early winter.

As time for graduation came, I was very pleased and proud of myself to learn that I was in the upper third of my class. Of my medical school class, there were 135 graduates. Forty-one became full professors.

When I got my MD degree in June of 1939 and started home to begin my internship in Rochester, I was extremely happy. It was the fulfillment of a long wish and hope that began all the way back in the fifth or sixth grade. I felt that my MD was something that nobody could take away from me.

INTERNSHIP

I reported to Strong Memorial for my surgical internship on July 1, 1939, and was immediately thrust into a completely different life. There is a traditional piece of advice to patients—never be admitted to the hospital on July 1 of any year because that is the time the new interns start, and they don't know much about what they are doing. There is some truth to this. My first duty was in the emergency room.

I had never done any work in the emergency room during medical school and I was not prepared for the type of cases that suddenly appeared. Of course, I had residents helping me. I had to learn to examine the trauma victim rapidly and make decisions rapidly about what was wrong and what to do. Within a few days, I had picked up the basics of what I needed to know.

Rochester was a peaceful city but a fairly sizable one; yet in thirteen weeks, I never saw a gunshot wound or a knife wound. That would be somewhat different now. We did have a lot of very severe automobile accident victims and the usual orthopedic problems involving broken bones.

I progressed to work on the wards. There the people became my own patients. I got to know them well. If the patient was operated on, I assisted in the operation. That is when I really began to learn surgical technique, and I did my best to improve. I kept some string in the intern quarters and spent any available moment of free time practicing tying knots. I also practiced with a surgical clamp. I would look away from something and then look back at it and quickly apply the clamp to a fold of a sheet or some other structure, so I gradually became more dexterous with the instruments.

My internship was challenging. We had quite a bit of night work and very little time off from duty. I figured that was why I was there—to learn. I learned a lot about human nature. Some of the ways people lived astonished me. I remember one instance in which I was treating a girl on the ward for inflammation of the pelvic organs due to acute gonorrhea. She told me she was engaged to the fellow who was coming to visit her in the hospital. One day, he stopped me on rounds and asked, "What is the matter with her?"

I asked her permission before I would tell him, and she readily consented. So, when he asked me again I said, "She has gonorrhea." I backed off, not knowing what reaction to expect.

His simply shrugged. "Well, that's what she gets for playing around."

I guess the engagement went on as before.

One of the advantages of training at Harvard compared to Strong was that, in Boston, I was educated in three hospitals, not just one. I might have a surgeon at one hospital tell me, "Everyone has to be operated for acute gallbladder disease," and then go to another hospital and be told "We don't operate on anyone with acute cholecystitis unless we wait for the inflamation to subside." In contrast, at Strong, the residents came through with one set of professors and sometimes believed there was only one way to do everything. However, there were some advantages to me from my time in Rochester. During the two years of surgical internship, I spent time on all the surgical specialty services including orthopedics, neurosurgery and genitourinary surgery. I have since looked back and recognized how extremely valuable this experience was because it gave me such a broad base for the medical career ahead. I not only learned some of the treatments for conditions addressed in these various specialties, but I also advanced my diagnostic skills. When patients later came to me in my gynecological practice, I found they frequently had a problem that involved other organ systems.

One of the major events of the two-year internship was that, after a year of courting, I married one of the operating room nurses, Betty Hunt.

When I started internship, I was ready to look for someone to date. Because of the work and night call, as well as limited financial resources, there had been very little opportunity for a social life in medical school. In Rochester, a friend I had known in both college and medical school was now with me in internship. One day in the operating room, he told Betty I was available for a date, although I had never met her. Telephone calls were exchanged, and soon a "blind date" was arranged.

The first time we went out, we joined the "matchmaker," Tom Smith, and his date for dinner and dancing at a place on the shore of Lake Ontario. We were in a convertible, and, by the time we arrived, Betty's hair had blown in every direction. I pointed out—probably unwisely—that it appeared that a crow had made a nest in her hair. The remark would come back to haunt me for more than 70 years! Nevertheless, we kept dating.

We got married September, 1940, at the First Presbyterian Church in Phelps. Her nearest relatives were in Canada, both her parents having died when she was a child—her mother died when Betty was four, and her father, when she was nine. In war time, it wasn't easy to travel or send gifts across the Canadian border, so we chose my hometown for the wedding.

Finances were a problem, but that was nothing new. There had not been any extra money all the way through the 1930s. Interns got nothing except their room and board, uniforms and laundry. Because nurses were paid $75 a month, plus room and board in the hospital nursing home, my bride and I managed. I was able to borrow a monthly sum from my older brother who by that time was fairly successful as treasurer of the Roebling Steel Company. With what he loaned me and what Betty made, and by eating most of our meals at the hospital, we were able to have a small attic apartment. There was not much expense for buying clothes because we didn't go out or entertain very much. We subsisted on about $100 cash a month.

I began to make plans to try and get an appointment at one of the hospitals in Boston for a residency. After submitting applications, I took a trip to Boston for an interview with Dr. Irving, then chief at Boston Lying-In Hospital and Professor of Obstetrics at Harvard. The interview went very well, and a month or two later I received word that I had been appointed. My internship at Strong Memorial in Rochester ended June 30, 1941.

RESIDENCY

I reported to work as a resident on August 1, 1941, at the Boston Lying-In Hospital—a great institution. It was completely under control of the medical school. There was a business executive superintendent in charge of the financial operation and administration, but Dr. Irving ran the professional side of the hospital and—I might add—ran it with an iron hand. He was known around the world as a very fine obstetrician who had done a great deal of research to make childbirth safer. It is interesting that when he took over as chief at the Lying-In, in the early 1930s, the maternal mortality rate at the hospital was about thirteen-per-thousand live births. He reduced it to about three-per-thousand live births at the time that I was a resident there.

Dr. Irving was the head of the big hospital with 5500 deliveries a year during my residency. One day he said to me, "Lew, when you are the head of an institution like this, every day you think you've seen the height of stupidity, and the next day you find you've only scratched the surface."

About 3500 of those 5500 women having babies were charity patients, cared for entirely by the house staff—the interns and residents. The other 2,000 or so were patients of the private obstetricians who had been appointed to the hospital medical staff. The house staff had very little to do with these patients except in emergencies or when they were asked by the visiting man to assist him in their care.

The number of deliveries made it a wonderful place to learn obstetrics because, since so many deliveries are perfectly normal, one has to perform a large number to encounter complications. Adding to our exposure to medical problems were the referrals of patients with complications from other hospitals in the area.

Many times in my obstetrical career, when I was holding a baby in my arms immediately after it was delivered, I would look down on it and marvel at the fact that a sperm and egg had gotten together and formed this extremely complex individual with everything in the right place and functioning well.

Partway through my residency at the Lying-In, I switched over to the Free Hospital—a wonderful place to learn GYN surgery—and then I was assigned back at the Lying-In for my final year. The war upset schedules and made it necessary for us to switch back and forth. Some of the residencies were depleted because men went into the Army and Navy after their first year. In addition, there also weren't as many visiting men to oversee the services and help the remaining house staff. It made a difference which draft board one was registered with. In Rochester, it was thought that physicians would be of more value to the military if they finished their training whereas in Boston, it wasn't unusual to be taken after a year of internship. I didn't change draft boards even though I moved from Rochester to Boston.

One of the great things about training at both the Boston Lying-In, which was predominantly for obstetrics, and the Free Hospital for Women, which was entirely for gynecology was that the visiting men, our instructors, almost never operated on clinic patients. Instead, they would help the resident do the operation. The resident was the surgeon for that case. This was good—the more challenging the procedures involved, the better. They would often let us do the case saying, "I'll help you." We wanted to do everything we could. Even Dr. Irving would come up from the academic offices to the clinical units to teach us and, on several occasions, would assist us in doing difficult procedures. In so many of the other residencies at that time, visiting men did most of the operating and residents only assisted.

The Free Hospital was under the strict direction of Harvard Medical School. It was started in the late 1800s by a group of wealthy society Bostonian women, and the chief gynecologist was a professor at Harvard Medical School. It was founded to take care of gynecologic problems of the poor classes in Boston, and it maintained its open access well past my residency. It influenced me. Part of its effect on me was the generosity of the founders, but a bigger part was seeing the reaction of the people when they learned they could receive care from top physicians in the country—free. The patients had one day a year they brought gifts—pies, towels, things they could afford—and they poured out their gratitude. We don't see it much today. The Free Hospital and the Boston Lying-In are now the top two floors of the Brigham and Women's Hospital.

Betty did not initially accompany me to Boston for two reasons: one was that I had to find a place for us to stay, and the other was that during the first month of the residency, I saw little rest. As the most junior man, I was responsible for delivering all the first babies—those of the "primiparas." Once a week I was off from 6 p.m. to midnight. The rest of the time, I was on call. I was glad to have the work, because that was what I was there for. I almost set the record for the most babies delivered by one resident in a month. The hospital record was 95. I delivered 94.

During the first month, I found a room for us in a rooming house near the hospital. When Betty joined me, we were both able to get our meals in the hospital. Betty tried working in two or three of the hospitals, but they were paying even less than they were in Rochester. The top operating nurses earned only $125 a month, without their room and board. So Betty finally went on private duty. In that way, she was somewhat able to control how much she worked.

We residents did our own laboratory work, even on private patients. Hospitals made good money off us. We did urinalyses, complete blood counts and other admission laboratory tests. We did crossmatches for blood transfusions. One of the big things that happened while I was at the Free Hospital was that, for the first time, residents got paid. The first income I made was $25 a month. Until then, we had received our uniforms, room and board, but that was all. Then suddenly, the Board of Directors at the hospital voted that we should be paid $25 a month. After a period of time, we learned the reason. The visiting surgeons at the hospital had complained to the board that some of the residents were always bumming cigarettes from them because they didn't have money to buy any. So, in order to give us the money to buy cigarettes, they paid us $25 a month. Because I didn't smoke, I was way ahead of the game. In those days, $25 went quite a ways.

Obstetrics

Having babies was quite different in the early 1940s. That was before the availability of antibiotics. We saw medical complications which were dangerous for the mother during pregnancy as well as for the baby. We had a large number of girls—a term commonly used for our female patients and not considered disrespectful in that day—with severe heart damage from rheumatic fever, which they usually had encountered in their early teens. There was research going on to determine the best way to take care of them. Most of them were Catholic; most would not have an abortion even if we told them of the possibility of losing their lives during the pregnancy. We had more maternal deaths from congestive heart failure during pregnancy than we did from actual obstetrical complications. We worked with a cardiologist who specialized in the care of pregnant women with heart disease. Because studies at that time showed that the total blood volume in pregnancy rises to a peak in the seventh month and then decreases after that point, we did not deliver the fetus at the time of the patient's distress—which would risk the life of both the mother and the baby—but treated her aggressively instead.

Chronic nephritis was another complication we had to deal with frequently. It was derived from various streptococcal infections our patients had as children, leaving their kidneys badly damaged. When women who were pregnant got pneumonia, it was a very serious—potentially life-threatening—situation. Most of these conditions are not seen anymore, at least not with such severity. Today antibiotics eradicate the underlying cause of the disease.

VAGINAL BIRTHS

Most of the first deliveries were done with what we called "outlet" forceps. As the baby came down the birth canal and was just about ready to deliver, the patient was put to sleep and we just lifted the baby out with forceps. Research showed that was better for the baby than having the mother push and push and push at that stage of the delivery. In addition, the fetal heart was very carefully monitored with a stethoscope so that if anything happened, such as a drop in the fetal heart rate, we would immediately deliver the baby.

Prolonged labor was dealt with differently from the way it is now. Patients were allowed to labor much longer than they are now. A woman really had to earn her cesarean section then. Labor of a day and a half to two days was not terribly unusual. Frequently, with the long labors, the contractions or "pains" weren't effective and not much was being accomplished until the end, when the patients would finally—after 12 to 14 hours—have a vaginal or "pelvic delivery." They were watched carefully and if the baby showed signs of problems or the mother became exhausted, we would instead do a cesarean section. This called for judgment.

CESAREAN SECTIONS

Fairly early in my career at the Lying-In, when I had been on a 12-hour night duty and had finally been able to go to the call room to get some sleep, hospital personnel woke me up about noon and said that there was a cesarean section to do. They said if I was willing to get up, the more senior physicians wanted me to do it. This would be my first cesarean section, so there wasn't any question that I was very happy to get up to do it, even though I hadn't slept much. The operation went well, and I was thrilled to have delivered my first cesarean baby.

We did a number of abdominal deliveries for misplaced placentas and placentas which separated early, causing heavy bleeding. We were trained to do cesareans in a short period of time. Always available was a "cesarean set up"—a tray with sterile instruments.

At the time, we did far fewer cesareans than are done now. Our cesarean section rate was down to about 2% as opposed to the greater-than 25% rate currently in many institutions. Cesareans were avoided except for extreme circumstances because they were not as safe then as they are now. Getting the mother through the delivery safely was the primary concern. There were several reasons why it was not as safe.

We had no antibiotics, so there was no way to treat a fulminating infection.

We had no blood banks at that time. The only way we could transfuse a patient was to have the family bring in a large number of relatives. We would draw blood on them and find a donor who would match. That was time-consuming, and in obstetrics, with the patient bleeding heavily while blood is being sought, it could intensify already difficult situations.

We didn't have very good anesthesia. The main anesthesia at the time was drop ether, which was relatively safe but very unpleasant for the patients. We did some spinal anesthesia, but it required someone who really knew what they were doing and there weren't many around with such qualifications. In extremely sick, desperately ill patients, we could do some cesareans under local anesthesia. It was a long and tedious task to inject an anesthetic liquid at multiple sites in the tissues to be incised.

BREECH

Nowadays, almost all babies in breech position, whether feet-first or buttocks first, are delivered by cesarean section. In contrast, during my residency and early practice years, women with breeches all started labor unless the pelvis was obviously too small. During the first examination of an obstetrical patient, we made a determination if the pelvis was of normal size or big or small. If the pelvis seemed to be normal, women with breeches were usually allowed to go into labor unless something else was wrong. For example, most of us found that if a labor progressed fairly rapidly and normally and the breech descended into the pelvis normally, it would be unlikely that there would be trouble delivering the baby through the vagina. If labor didn't progress well, or the breech didn't descend well into the pelvis, it was time to consider doing a cesarean. Of course, there were risks when delivering any breech through the pelvis. Although we delivered most of them safely, we occasionally got into trouble and wished we hadn't proceeded with a plan for a vaginal birth. Several things could happen. The membranes might rupture, and if the fetus did not fill the pelvic space, the umbilical cord could prolapse, dropping ahead of the baby. A part of the baby could press on the cord and cut off the blood supply. Therefore, the patient with a breech had to be monitored very carefully by stethoscope during labor to assure that the fetal heart rate was perfectly normal.

Because the baby's head was the biggest part of the baby and it came out last, if we got the rest of the baby out and the head was too big, we were faced with great difficulty. Occasionally, we needed to put forceps on the after-coming head. This was not too difficult to do. The usual forceps could be used for that, but Dr. Piper in Philadelphia developed special breech-delivery forceps, which were angled differently and seem to fit better. (In those days, procedures, equipment and diseases were frequently given the name of the one who introduced them.) In order to get the Piper forceps on correctly, we had to kneel on the floor and get our head and shoulders down to the correct level to insert them into the vagina and apply them around the head. We came to learn that perhaps the attitude of prayer was for a very good reason.

When a breech was detected before the patient went into labor, for example, at eight months or so, we might attempt to turn the baby. This could be an extremely difficult affair and uncomfortable for the patient. We were taught to get a hold of the baby through the abdominal wall. With one hand we would grasp the head and press in one direction and with the other hand we would grasp the baby's rump and press in the other direction, gradually shifting the fetus around to where the head was down and the buttocks up. But it didn't always work. In fact, frequently we would get stuck partway around and would have to push the baby back. Sometimes after we had worked and worked and got the baby turned around, the baby would immediately turn itself back the other way. Seeing that babies could rotate themselves a lot easier than I could, I never found turning breeches a useful procedure. Nowadays, medications are used to relax the uterine muscle, making the procedure more successful and more comfortable, although not risk-free.

Another fetal "malposition" we encountered was a baby being carried in a transverse lie—that is, lying crosswise in the uterus. The head would be on one side and buttocks on the other. If the fetus resisted very gentle turning, this was almost a 100% indication for a cesarean section.

MULTIPLE PREGNANCIES

In one case, all of us—including The Professor—were completely fooled. The patient had considerable toxemia. Toxemia is a condition of high blood pressure with pregnancy that encompasses both preeclampsia and eclampsia. In her case, it was not life-threatening. She had been in the hospital for about three weeks to stabilize her condition. Each day, accompanied by Dr. Irving, we checked on her status, and as she got better from the toxemia, we started to talk about inducing labor because she was obviously at term. It was advisable to conclude the pregnancy because of the toxemia. However, we were not sure of her due date, because her uterus was considerably bigger than her menstrual dates would have warranted. We could feel the baby perfectly well through the abdominal wall, and it seemed plenty large. Since some people menstruate for a month or two after they are pregnant, there could simply be a dating discrepancy. Every time we started talking about inducing labor she kept saying, "I'm not ready. I'm not ready."

We said, "Nonsense, the baby is big at seven to eight pounds from feeling of it." Dr. Irving concurred that it was certainly ready. Finally, over her objections, we convinced her to go ahead and induce labor, which went very smoothly, except that once she delivered her baby, she presented us with another. The twins—that not one of us had diagnosed—were over 6 pounds each. Of course, in the 1940s, there weren't sonograms, and we didn't think it necessary to do an X-ray because it was so "obvious" that she only had one baby.

I was the envy of some of the other residents at Lying-In Hospital, because I delivered two sets of triplets. Triplets, before the use of fertility drugs, came on an average of one set in every 7,700 deliveries. So, not many people had delivered them. The first set that I delivered was for a woman who had attended our prenatal clinic. Her three babies were of tremendous size for triplets. They weighed 7 ½ pounds apiece. The babies and the placenta weighed 24 pounds together. This was quite a load for her to carry around. The delivery went very well. The babies all delivered through the pelvis and were in excellent condition. A cesarean would probably have been done today. Since she was unmarried, the hospital did its best to keep the birth quiet. However, about the second day of her postpartum period, newspeople and photographers arrived and demanded to see the babies and take pictures of them. The hospital found that she had called the newspapers herself about it. It didn't make any difference to her that she was single. She wanted the notoriety of it, and with triplets, baby food companies gave a free one-year supply, and diaper companies gave free diapers.

My patient with the second set of triplets, was only about 4 ½ months pregnant when she went into labor, and of course, those babies did not live. Later in my private practice, I was called into consultation and delivered another set of triplets, this time at 7 ½ months' gestation. All three lived and did fine.

OBSTETRIC TRAGEDIES

One day, when I was running the outpatient department for a home-delivery district, I examined a woman whose fetus was beginning to become hydrocephalic—the baby was starting to accumulate intracranial fluid inside the brain. I felt the relatively large head palpable over the pubic bone and sent her for an X-ray. She was admitted to the hospital and treated. I got some commendation for the early diagnosis from both the visiting man and The Professor. They were amazed that I diagnosed it so early. I didn't think it was all that clever.

I remember my last delivery at the Lying-In in 1943. The management of it demonstrates a striking contrast to the way obstetrics is practiced now. On a Tuesday we had admitted, a primipara in labor with a terrible horror story. She had been an inpatient at a small coastal hospital north of Boston since the previous Saturday afternoon. She was in labor with her first baby. The fetal head was very high, not engaged in the pelvis, a situation in which no attempt should be made to deliver her, but someone at the referral hospital had tried to do a "high-forceps procedure" and managed to get the instruments up into the uterine cavity. It was fortunate that he didn't tear part of the uterus in the process. One rule of obstetrics that must never be broken is, "Never apply forceps to a head not in the pelvis."

He couldn't pull the baby down into the pelvis, so he took the forceps off and put her back to bed and let her labor some more. This was a terrible mistake, because he had inevitably induced infection into the uterus with the attempt at delivery. She labored through the weekend, and on Monday morning, another doctor at the same hospital tried again to deliver her with high forceps. The head was still not in the pelvis and couldn't be pulled in. So again the forceps were removed and she was put back to bed. Finally, on Tuesday noon, she was sent into the Lying-In by ambulance. When she arrived, she had a temperature of 104° and a pulse of over 160 beats per minute. She was desperately ill, and the baby's head was still out of the pelvis. Furthermore, the baby had died after all the manipulation at the other hospital.

It was felt that it was much too dangerous to try to do a cesarean section because we didn't have good antibiotics, and by taking the baby out through the abdomen, we would certainly give her peritonitis, which could be lethal. So, the attending obstetrician told me to deliver her the best way I could. I got a hand up into the uterus and assessed the situation. It was a very large baby and a very large head that wouldn't come down into the pelvis. I placed one hand on the head to act as a guide, and with the other, I inserted a large, very heavy pair of long-handled scissors and cut a hole in the scalp and skull and evacuated the brains. This collapsed the head. The smaller diameter allowed me to pull the baby's head into the pelvis. I could get the collapsed head down into the vagina, but I could not get the shoulders; the shoulders were too big. So again, under extremely challenging conditions with an intricate situation, using one hand inside the uterus as a guide on the baby, I managed to pass some scissors up there with the other hand and cut both clavicles. This action collapsed the shoulders somewhat. I could then get the shoulders into the upper pelvis, but I couldn't get the abdomen or the chest. So for a third time I went back with the heavy scissors, cut the ribs and evacuated the chest. I was then, with some difficulty, able to pull the baby down into the vagina and deliver it.

The baby was so large that the portion I delivered, weighed 11 ½ pounds! Despite the success of avoiding the dangerous abdominal surgery, we were not sure the woman was going to make it because of her severe infection. Fortunately, all of these manipulations had not damaged her uterus, and after a stormy course, she survived. This was the first time I had ever done anything of that magnitude. I was horrified by the patient's tragedy but also proud of the fact that the visiting man let me do the procedure in such a highly complex situation.

OBSTETRIC STORIES

Thankfully, the serious things that happened on the delivery floor were also interspersed with things that, in retrospect, lightened up the day a bit.

We had medical students delivering women who already had several babies—six, seven, eight or more. One day, while I was coaching a student, all of the anesthetists were busy, so I had to give the anesthesia and teach at the same time. In those days, the woman's feet were put up in stirrups and drapes were routinely put over the legs and across the abdomen. After the patient was asleep, a towel was clipped across from the sheet draping one buttock to the sheet draping the other. The purpose was to keep the anus covered so that there was less chance of bacteria entering the field where the baby would emerge. This student got his gown and was ready. I had been giving the patient drop ether. In order to see what the student was doing, I had knelt up on the delivery table with the patient's head between my knees so I could look over her abdomen to see what the student was doing.

I could tell the student was extremely nervous. The baby was ready to deliver with the next pain, but I had the patient pretty deep so she couldn't push. So I told the student to get ready and I would put gentle pressure on the abdomen. "Are you ready?" I said.

"Yes," he said, and stood there with his hands up.

I gave a good push on the abdomen, and because she had delivered seven or eight babies before, the baby came out very rapidly with the head moving upward, almost as if it were coming off a ski jump. The student never moved a muscle; he was completely frozen. The baby disappeared between her legs, and I thought, Oh, God, the baby's fallen on the floor.

I jumped off the head of the table, ran around and looked down on the floor. The baby wasn't there. I looked up and saw the baby had caught between the patient's buttocks and the towel. The newborn had slid down behind the towel up to his armpits and was hanging with his head above, both arms over and body behind the towel. He was just kind of swinging there, oblivious to my sense of great relief.

One day, I was just outside the labor room door when a student nurse came rushing out. She had panic in her voice. "I can't hear the fetal heart on this patient anymore!" I ran in. The patient was a very large woman. I pulled down the sheet on the bed to quickly assess the situation. Her abdomen looked flatter than it should, in spite of the obesity. I lowered the sheet further to find the baby was sitting down between her knees on the bed.

We enjoyed teaching the medical students, remembering we were once the recipients of the residents' mentoring. In those days, the way that we estimated the labor progress was by doing a rectal examination. We could press the anterior wall of the rectum and feel the cervix against the fetal head. We determined how much she was dilated by estimating finger breadths. By doing a rectal we didn't have to invade the vagina, avoiding the risk of introducing bacteria. Now obstetricians do vaginal exams; it has proven to be safe.

I examined a woman while trying to teach the students about rectal exams. I turned around to the student and told him where the cervix was and where he could find it upon exam. "She's two fingers dilated," I explained, meaning that the distance across the open cervix was estimated to be that of two finger breadths. "You go ahead and examine her now," I said. To convey to the student a sense of responsibility, I added, "I'll be out in the hall."

Immediately after I stepped out, I heard screams from the labor room. I thought, Gosh, she can't be delivering now! I went back again to see what the matter was.

The student was standing by the bed chagrined. He said, "I don't know how you can say this patient is two fingers dilated; I can't get two fingers in her rectum."

It's a good thing I hadn't told him she was four fingers dilated.

The front door of the hospital was an entrance for patients in labor. On one side was a counter where a receptionist sat and behind the counter was the telephone operator at an old-fashioned switchboard. One night, a highway patrol car wheeled into the driveway and up to the front door with screeching brakes and a screaming siren. A highway patrolman's wife down on Cape Cod, 70 miles away, had developed premature labor pains at about seven months' gestation. He came roaring up to

Boston and drove up to the hospital front doors. He came rushing in extremely excited. Without waiting, he vaulted the reception desk counter and grabbed the telephone operator by the shoulders and started yelling, "Get a doctor! Get a doctor!" He was shaking the poor woman so hard she couldn't plug in any of the wires.

I happened to be coming down the hall at just that moment. I heard all this commotion and ran in to see what was going on. I heard his shouts and saw the problem .I rushed out and down the steps and to the car and opened the door of the police car where his wife was sitting in the front seat. She looked okay. I said, "Are you all right?"

"Yes, I'm fine," she said, "but please go in there and do something about my husband."

After getting him calmed down, we got her admitted, and things went well with her preterm problem.

One night when I was on duty, a taxi drove up to the back patient entrance with a woman in labor. The driver rushed in and said to "get somebody out here." I went out to find a very large lady in the back seat moaning and groaning. I pulled up her dress to see what was going on. She had on a pair of very large black bloomers that went from the upper abdomen to just above the knees. I tugged on the top elastic to assess the situation and, to my surprise, encountered a newborn baby. It had been born earlier and was nestled down in the crotch of the bloomers. We had a sterile tray under the desk for situations like this. I simply clamped the cord, cut it, extracted the baby from the bloomers, dropped the cord back into the bloomers and let the elastic snap back. I had the driver take her around to the patient entrance where we could get her on a stretcher up to the delivery room and deliver the placenta.

There was a rumor at the time about a woman who had delivered on the grounds of the hospital in a car. When the bill came, it included the cost of use of a delivery room. The husband went down to the superintendent of the hospital and objected to the charge, since his wife hadn't been in the delivery room. The story is that the superintendent said, "Okay," crossed out the delivery room charge and wrote "greens fee" on it.

We had a wing of the hospital that was devoted to a nurses' dormitory, where the student nurses and the single private-duty nurses lived. The superintendent of nurses also lived there. She was an older single woman. In those days, the early days of World War II, the traffic was heavy and the trains were very crowded and often late. She had a close friend in New York City who was coming up to spend the weekend with her. The traveler had arranged a specific time to be at the Lying-In to meet the schedule of her friend, the super of nurses. They were planning on doing something special late in the afternoon. The train came into the South Station in Boston, which is quite a way from the hospital. But the train from New York was quite late, making it problematic to meet the agreed-upon time. She disembarked as rapidly as possible, collected her bag, rushed out, got into a taxi and said, "Go to the Boston Lying-In and get there as quick as you can!"

The taxi driver rose to the occasion and started weaving in and out of traffic, going through the streets faster than the speed limit. He got out on one of the freeways, and an officer on a motorcycle drove up next to him and put on his siren to pull him over for going so fast. The driver opened his window and yelled, "I am going to the Lying-In."

That is all the officer needed to hear. He yelled back with a great sense of importance, "Follow me!" He gunned up ahead of the taxi, put on his siren and went roaring to the Lying-In, providing a motorcycle escort.

When they got there, the passenger got out, thanked the driver, paid her fee and walked into the hospital to meet her friend, much to the amazement of both the driver and the police officer.

One Christmas morning when I was on the obstetrics service at Lying-In, a service man's wife was in labor. He had just been brought home from the army. I went to tell him he had a nice baby boy. That big burly uniformed soldier stared at me and then collapsed on the floor.

Gynecology

The Free Hospital was a small hospital with probably fewer than 100 beds. It did have a wing where the attending surgeons could bring their private patients. None of the ward patients paid for their care. It was amazing to see the gratitude of the women. When a patient came to the outpatient department for any sort of gynecological complaint and was seen by one of the residents or a visiting doctor, if it were decided that something needed to be done surgically, she would be scheduled for the operation, regardless of whether it was for benign tumors, cancer, radium insertion for carcinoma of the cervix or an infertility operation.

The outpatients had an infertility clinic under the direction of Dr. John Rock, a nationally known expert and one of the two men who together developed the birth control pill. During the 1940s, he and Dr. Marshall Hertig, Professor of Pathology, developed a system that contributed greatly to the knowledge of early embryos. If a woman needed a hysterectomy and was of childbearing age, they would instruct her regarding her fertility time and would then schedule the operation for a certain number of days after expected ovulation. She was encouraged to have intercourse during the fertility time and then come into the hospital. The surgeons would tie off the Fallopian tubes and wash out the lower abdomen before removing the uterus. After the surgery, the researchers would carefully go over the tubes and the uterus in search of any early fertilized ovum. The conceptus, possibly retrieved as early as 48-hours after conception, could then be studied to see how life started. This greatly advanced the science of early pregnancy. They found some specimens—called blastocysts—of only four or eight cells.

The Free Hospital had two operating rooms set up very efficiently. There was a small anesthesia room right outside the two rooms. Toward the end of an operation, one of the two scrub nurses would drop out, re-scrub and get the instruments for the next operation ready over at one side of the operating room. Then one of the anesthetists would put the next patient to sleep in the small room outside so that, when one operation was finished, another could begin almost immediately. Because of concern about cross contamination, this would not be the way it would be done now, but in those days, we believed we were being careful about the sterility.

The resident would go out into the dressing room and quickly dictate the operative report for the medical record, and by the time he got back in and was scrubbed, the next patient was in the suite with her operation ready to start. Consequently, we were able to go through a fairly sizable schedule. Usually we started operating about 6:15 in the morning and finished about 1:30 or 2:00 in the afternoon.

The operating rooms were not air conditioned. No place in the hospital was air-conditioned. We would perspire almost through our gowns, and we always had one extra nurse in the operating room who did nothing but wipe the sweat from the foreheads of the surgical team so that it wouldn't fall into the incision. Sometimes we had to change all of our undergarments between operations because they were soaking wet by the time we finished.

The operating room nurses were highly skilled. They were a great help to the residents in the early stages of their surgical training. Occasionally, if I was not entirely sure how to attack a problem or what to do next, I could hold out my hand for an instrument and see what the scrub nurse would put in it. As a consequence of the excellent operating nurses and the experience granted by the visiting men and the variety and number of patients, everyone who finished residency at the Free Hospital was a highly trained and very polished surgeon.

One of our surgery educators was Dr. Frank Pemberton. He was Professor of Gynecology at Harvard and Chief of Staff at the Free Hospital and was responsible for a lot of good research that was going on there at the time. He was a very fast surgeon and talked in a high, squeaky voice.

He was very tense while he was operating. Every resident assisting him tried to get through the operation without being fussed at, but nobody ever did. He didn't really mean anything by his grousing, but he kept up a steady line of complaint. He wanted everything "just so" on the assisting end. We had to keep all the blood away from the field and we had to try and stay ahead of him. He would constantly be fussing, "C'mon, c'mon. Good God! Haven't you ever seen an operation before? Try to be some help, will ya? Try to be some help!"

And if we asked a question about something, he would likely say, "Shouldn't talk while you're operating."

One of my experiences was to operate with Dr. Pemberton at the American College of Surgeons meeting when it was in Boston one year. People attending the conference would go to different hospitals and watch famous surgeons operate. Dr. Pemberton called me to assist him while he did one of those demonstrations.

There was a bank of seats arranged at the head of the operating table, which was on a riser, and the patient was tilted head-down so the visitors could see in the wound. I knew all those doctors were up there watching.

We started in. Dr. Pemberton was operating with his head down, working fast, and I was doing my best to keep up and doing it well. He started his usual, "C'mon, C'mon. Haven't you seen that before? Good God! Be some help, will ya?" Then he'd raise his head up and for the benefit of the observers, he would say in a very fine voice, "See how we do this and how well it goes?"

Then he would look down again and say to me, "Ouch! Damn it! Be some help will ya?" In a few minutes, after ranting in a very low voice, he would turn to the audience and say how well it was going.

He had the same scrub nurse all the time. He treated the scrub nurses better than he treated the doctor—his lowly assistant. The residents were beneath him.

He was very set in his ways. He always liked to have the tissue forceps he used in one specific spot on the instrument tray. One day, I had picked up his forceps to hold a piece of the bowel out of the way for him, and without looking, he reached to get his forceps, and they weren't there. They were down in the incision. When he saw where they were and that they weren't where he wanted them, instead of asking me for them, he turned to the scrub nurse and said, "He's got my forceps. Get them and give them to me!" So I gave them to her and she gave them to him.

It is reminiscent of a situation a colleague told me about, in which a surgeon's similar behavior backfired. An assistant resident working under me told me of an experience he had when he started his surgery rotation.

Residents at Harvard were required to have at least two years of surgery training before being accepted in the residency. He was obtaining his during an internship at Beth Israel in New York. Operations for hernia repair under local anesthesia were just starting up. The visiting man was helping him do his first hernia repair under local anesthesia. The patient was wide awake. He wasn't doing things the way the attending physician wanted him to. The visiting man kept interrupting, talking, correcting, telling him how to do it right, saying to the intern, "Oh, no! Not that way, do it this way! No, no, not like that!"

He continued criticizing until finally, the patient, cognizant of everything that was happening, said, "Doctor, if he makes you so nervous, why don't you do it yourself?"

Family Planning

Teaching hospitals were interested in promoting birth control for large families. During my residency, the only birth control method we had to offer was the diaphragm. We had a clinic where women could come in and be fitted for a diaphragm and be taught to use it. One afternoon a week, I worked in a special diaphragm clinic. This was quite an education in the sex lives of people. I had to ask specific questions like, "How often do you have sex?" I did an examination, and if everything was okay, I fitted a diaphragm and instructed the woman how to use it. She was taught how to put it in and take it out and was advised to take a douche the next morning after it was removed.

After I showed one patient how to use her new diaphragm, she put it in correctly, took it out, got down off the table and said, "This ain't going to work."

I said, "What do you mean? You know how to do it, and it will work all right if you use it."

She said, "No, I never knows what time my husband's coming home, and once he puts his hand on the doorknob, I ain't got time to do all this!"

Another woman said, "I have intercourse every night."

I gently offered advice. "Put the diaphragm in every night and take it out in the morning."

She said, "What shall I do if we have intercourse in the morning?"

I said, "You already told me you had intercourse every night. How often do you have intercourse in the morning?"

She said, "Well, most every time we has it at night we has it again in the morning."

I ended up telling her to try to find some time during the day to take it out and douche before putting it back in.

Dr. Eastman, Professor of Obstetrics at John Hopkins, had a program designed to control family size in poor people. The standing policy on the obstetrical unit was that all women having their first babies were admitted to the hospital. His program offered an exception. Any woman who had delivered at least three babies and who wanted a tubal ligation could also come into the hospital and have her baby. This incentive program occasionally backfired. Some women would say that they were going to have a tubal ligation. They would come in and have their baby in the hospital; then when it was time to do the ligation the next day after the delivery, they would say that they had decided not to have it. So they got a free hospital delivery without having the sterilization procedure.

Research

There was always interesting research going on at the hospitals. Almost everybody was interested in cancer, which sparked my interest. Some researchers at the hospital were studying eclampsia and preeclampsia—pregnancy conditions associated with high blood pressure, fluid retention, protein in the urine and, in the case of eclampsia, seizures.

There was a lot of research going on as to what was the best pain reliever during labor. We did all sorts of combinations of drugs, most of which produced "twilight sleep," in which the woman is sedated but not anesthetized—she is pretty much unaware of what is going on around her. In that day and age that was what the patients wanted. I think a private obstetrician would not have had much practice if he tried to get his patients to have natural childbirth. They would come into the hospital and some of them, as they were admitted, would start yelling, "Give me the needle! Give me the needle!" Natural childbirth was the last thing any of the women wanted at that time. When Demerol came on the market, we did research on whether or not it was safe for the mother for the pain of labor and safe for the baby before it was born.

During my residency, we started doing research on a new, promising medicine named "penicillin." When penicillin came out for clinical use, there was very little known about it. Because it was so promising, there was a great clamor for it. Everybody wanted it, and doctors were treating everything with it. But there was a very small supply. I believe that the government acted very sensibly in response. Dr. Chester Keefer, a Professor of Medicine at Boston University, was made the czar for all the penicillin in the country. He controlled every bit of it and doled it out to institutions for certain types of research to see what it would do for infections in various doses. Up until then, it wasn't known what the right dose would be. In 1942, he gave us a supply at the Lying-In for the treatment of mastitis, infection of the breast after delivery and breast abscesses—my first contact with penicillin.

Antibiotics changed medicine. Two professors had set their careers on learning everything there was to know about syphilis. For eight years they had worked to gather that information for a textbook. The month after their book came out, new antibiotics completely eradicated the disease, and the book was obsolete.

In my last year of residency, I went to Baltimore for a month at Johns Hopkins. A resident in that program came to Harvard at the same time and assumed my duties. Hopkins had obstetrical patients in large wards, as many as 40 women in a ward. There was a beautiful tradition there. Every Sunday morning, after the clinical treatments were over and the wards quieted down, one of the women would begin to sing spirituals. All the other patients joined in. I loved to pause in my work and listen each week.

When I finished my time at the Free Hospital and went back to the Lying-In, I faced my final year of training. As a senior resident, I was entrusted with some of the more difficult cases and had the opportunity to work with top visiting men and Dr. Irving. Some of the happiest times of my life were at the Lying-In and the Free Hospital for Women. I was doing what I wanted to do, something I had looked forward to since boyhood.

3

WORLD WAR II MILITARY SERVICE

I was the only doctor on the ship. After years of training to take care of women, here I was with three hundred men. Previously trying to find out what was the matter with new patients, I now had to determine whether anything was the matter with them at all, because too often, they tried to get out of work by coming down with various aches, pains and illnesses.

One day an excitable Italian boy came in complaining of a very severe backache. We had no X-ray capabilities. I treated him with various pain relievers, but he didn't get any better. I decided to inject some Novocain around the sacroiliac region and see if it would relax the muscles in the area and, in turn, relieve the pain.

I did not anticipate that he was deathly afraid of needles. As I prepared a syringe of Novocain, he made such a fuss, I had to have three corpsmen hold him down for the needle insertion. All the time he was screaming and carrying on. When he finally left, he told of his adventures to the other crewmen. The needle kept getting bigger and bigger. It was several months before anyone else complained of back pain, and my Italian friend did not return.

I went back to the Boston Lying-In for almost another year of residency and more learning. In November and early December, 1943, when I was well into my residency at the Boston Lying-In, there began to be pressure placed on people my age and physicians like me to get into the armed services. The draft board was willing to allow me to stay until I finished the complete residency, which would have been July, 1944, but I became eager to be part of what was going on, and friends were leaving for the military all the time. I talked to Dr. Irving and told him that I thought maybe it was up to me to get into the service and do my part. He agreed. Part of the agreement may have been because his young son, who was college age, had just gone into the army. I decided to enter the Navy Medical Corps on January 1, 1944. My papers were processed in Boston, and I was ready to go when I finished at the Lying-In on December 31, 1943.

I started out as a lieutenant junior grade, as was true of all doctors entering the Navy. On a certain date, after a year or so, they put out an order and all lieutenant JGs became full lieutenants.

In the Navy, a whole new group of experiences and a whole new group of things to learn awaited me My first assignment was to report to Kittery, Maine, just across the Piscataqua River from Portsmouth, New Hampshire. It was bitter cold up there the first of January.

The physicians did not live on the base. I found a room in a house in Portsmouth and every morning in zero-degree weather had to walk across the long bridge over the river to get to my duty. The base was building submarines. They had a 22,000-civilian workforce turning out about three submarines a month. There was a large U. S. Marine contingent. A group of marines, who had just been brought back from Guadalcanal, policed the submarine base and acted as guards for a Navy prison on the grounds.

My job was to work in the infirmary, which took care of not only the outpatient Navy personnel but also the civilians who might be injured on the job. This was new and interesting work. I had to learn to do things like dig small pieces of steel out of corneas.

I was at the base for about three months when I was ordered to a ship—a PT tender. It was being built in Baltimore. It would be the mothership of three squadrons of PTs in the South Pacific. The ship was being constructed on the hull of an LST—a landing ship tank. The LST is flat on the bottom and doesn't have much draft so that it can go up on the beach, open up the big front doors and the tanks can roll out. This was being modified so that the tank deck became large machine and carpentry shops where they took care of the PTs. There was a derrick on the side of the ship so that a PT to be worked on could be lifted out of the water. Despite being small craft, the PTs were fairly complicated. They were about 40 feet long, and they had two 12-cylinder Rolls Royce engines that gave a speed of about 35 knots. However, when they were fully armed and carrying several torpedoes, they were weighed down some and couldn't attain those speeds.

We were stationed in Baltimore while they finished the ship. Most of the wives—including my own—did not remain at Baltimore, knowing that we would be there for only two or three days. Betty and I had encountered some problems getting pregnant for which we had received help from Dr. Rock. My wife was four months pregnant when I sailed from Norfolk on June 4, 1944.

We started out for the South Pacific quite early that Sunday morning. We went in convoy. When we had been at sea only two days, we heard that the Normandy invasion had started. This was good news. It meant that we were that much closer, hopefully, to defeating Germany and the war would be over that much sooner. It would free up more forces to help in the Pacific. We all wanted to get it over and come home.

After we had left Norfolk, we rounded Cape Hatteras, which usually had a pretty good-sized sea running and was quite rough. The ship rolled badly and immediately we started having a large group of seasick new sailors. At least 50% of our crew—so-called boots—had not been to sea before. It was a really nice day, and those who were not on duty somewhere collected on deck to get the fresh air and, hopefully, to help the queasiness. We had a cook on board who had been on a destroyer, so he was not seasick. This seaman from the galley came out . . . I can still see him . . . overweight with a couple of days' growth of beard and wearing a greasy apron. He would come up to those who were trying not to be sick, pull out a plug of tobacco and bite off a big chew. Everybody would head for the rail. He delighted in doing that.

A few of the seasick men never got over the "distress." One of the chief engineers sat in the engine room with a pail beside him as long as he was on the ship. Later, as soon as we got enough control of the enemy, the Navy started letting the men with chronic seasickness go home. I was fortunate never to suffer from seasickness—in the war and to this day.

We were in convoy with some destroyers, mostly merchant ships. When we went through the Panama Canal, we found it to be heavily fortified as one would expect in wartime.

After we cleared the canal, we headed out into the Pacific. After we left the Panama Canal, we no longer had the convoy escort; we were completely alone. I enjoyed being on the sea. There was really not much danger once we cleared the Panama Canal because there weren't any German or Japanese submarines in those areas, and it was more or less clear sailing.

Our first stop was a coaling area on Bora Bora, an island about 90 miles from Tahiti. The ship made about eight knots per hour, so we were in for a long voyage. We had eighteen officers, all reservists except for two warrant officers who had come up through the ranks; there were no regular Navy officers on board. The captain of the ship was a lieutenant who had held a prior command on a small yacht-like-ship that patrolled outside of Newport. The executive officer was a contractor from Long Island. Of course, all the officers had been to special schools and were trained in what they were supposed to do.

There was quite a bit of card playing, including some bridge. I played a great deal of bridge. I never could get into poker. Some of the officers were good poker players and others were not but played for something to do. We had payday the first of the month. Most men allocated a certain amount of money for the month—such as $50—and when that was gone, would stop playing until the next payday. Most of the money ended up in the hands of a couple of very fine gamblers. One of them was one of the warrant officers who had come up through the regular Navy. The other was not an officer, just a highly-trained college graduate who was mathematically inclined. He knew the exact odds of coming up a certain number on every roll of dice and made a lot of money shooting craps. This officer would send home a couple of thousand dollars every so often. We were hit, and he was killed on the 29th of December that year, but before Christmas, he had sent home $2,000 from his gambling for his wife to buy a mink coat.

I was the only doctor on the ship. We had a crew of three hundred—all men, of course. After spending a great deal of time training to take care of women, here I was with three hundred men to take care of. I soon learned that whereas I had been used to seeing new patients and trying to find out what was the matter with them, in the Navy I first had to determine whether anything was the matter with them at all, because too often, they tried to get out of work by coming down with various aches, pains and illnesses.

One day an excitable Italian boy came in complaining of a very severe backache. I had not had a great deal of experience with back pain. We had no X-ray capabilities. I treated him with various pain relievers and other interventions for several days, and he didn't get any better. I decided to inject some Novocain where it was hurting around the sacroiliac region and see if it would relax the muscles in the area and, in turn, relieve the pain.

I did not anticipate that he was deathly afraid of needles. When I had him lie on his stomach as I prepared a syringe of Novocain, he made such a fuss I had to have three corpsmen hold him down for the needle insertion. All the time he was screaming and carrying on. When he finally got up and left, he began to tell of his adventures to the other crewmen. The needle kept getting bigger and bigger. The whole procedure was explained in the worst possible way. It was several months after that before anyone else complained of back pain, and my Italian friend did not return.

The relatively large two-room sick bay was below the main deck. One room had four beds, toilet facilities and an area for some nursing procedures. Across the hall was the examining room, which served as a small laboratory. We could only do a few laboratory tests, including complete blood counts and urinalyses. There were sterilizers for instruments and a table that would serve as both an examining table and, if necessary, an operating table. This is where I saw patients every morning. Patients came at about 8:30 a.m. We had a sick call, so to speak.

There were four corpsmen who had been medically trained. One was a chiropractor, one, a lawyer who worked for the government, one, a funeral director at a funeral home in a small town outside of Indianapolis and one, a boy about 18 years old who had finished high school and gone into the Navy where he had been trained as a corpsman. They were all very congenial fellas, and I got along with them very well. Their work was adequate, but I would have hated to have to do much real surgery with them.

There was no general anesthesia so anything we had to do was under local or spinal. There was a pharmacy stocked with quite a few drugs. Of course, we had no penicillin or other antibiotics at that time but we had the usual medications for pain, gastrointestinal upsets and other common complaints, although some of the drugs were long outdated and useless. We worked with what we had.

Dealing with the enlisted men was a new experience for me. I had seen fairly uneducated people in my residency and in my medical school practice, but I wasn't prepared for some of the things that I saw and still don't really understand. For instance, each of the lifeboats and life rafts on the ship had a first aid box on it with all sorts of emergency supplies in it, including morphine serettes. In inspecting those after having been at sea for some time, I found that all of the serettes of morphine in all of the first aid boxes had been stolen. I couldn't believe that someone could be dumb enough to steal what he may find a great need for in the near future. Such short-sightedness was incredible to me.

Partway across the Pacific on the way to New Guinea, we crossed the equator. There was a celebration on board, indoctrinating those of us who had never been across the equator before, into the office of Neptune.

I've always liked water, so I really enjoyed being on the ocean. When I wasn't busy, I would stand on deck and watch the flying fish go over the bow of the ship, glide a little distance and then dive back in.

I still remember how beautiful it was on deck in the South Pacific. The nights were wonderful in the starlight and moonlight. Because we were traveling completely blacked out, the stars were brilliant overhead. It was as though I could reach out and touch them. The Southern Cross was up where we could see it all the time. It had a religious significance to some of us. We felt as though we were being watched over whenever it was out there.

We, of course, had some storms which were very uncomfortable. The ship was flat-bottomed to allow it to get into relatively shallow water, and consequently it rolled excessively in any sort of heavy sea. This would toss me about if I was walking. If I was trying to sleep, it could bang me around in the bunk. If I was trying to eat, it could become difficult, with plates sliding everywhere.

Upon arriving at Bora Bora, we took on more oil. Bora Bora is about 2000 miles southwest of Honolulu. It is a single island. An extinct volcano forms a mountain in the middle of it, and, according to two people who did the navigation, we should have seen it about six a.m. on the morning of our planned arrival. At six, the ship sailed on and we had not yet seen it. Having been at sea 20 or 30 days without seeing land, and realizing that a very small degree of error in navigation could put us 100 miles one side or the other of a destination, there was some consternation on the bridge. They steamed on and kept checking the sextant—a navigation aid. Finally, about eight o'clock in the morning, to everyone's relief, the mountain showed up on the horizon.

Bora Bora was an island paradise, a beautiful place with a big coral reef surrounding it and a quiet bay inside. The islanders were the only people we saw, natives who looked like those in Dorothy Lamour movies. The French owned the place, and we were there on the 14th of July—Bastille Day. They held special events. Girls came out in their grass skirts and performed dances which were quite wild.

We left Bora Bora for Port Moresby, New Guinea, where we arrived two or three weeks later—sometime in August. New Guinea is a very large island. Port Moresby had been secured by MacArthur's troops some time before. MacArthur's strategy, after he had crossed from Australia into the eastern end of New Guinea and taken Port Moresby, was to leapfrog up the coast and make a landing, usually at a native village. His men would push the "Japs"—as the enemy troops were called then—back into the jungle, hold a ten-mile perimeter line and make an airstrip down by the beach. They would then use that airstrip to make another sortie up the coast and establish another airfield. When they got to an island that had a big bay and a very fine port, they established a very sizable base there to serve as one of the springboards for taking off for the Philippines.

So, we were to leapfrog by boat up the coast to pick up the PTs we were being assigned to manage. The first place we dropped anchor was Finchhaven.

At Finchhaven, things were pretty crude. There was an army camp there. As was typical, there was a ten-mile perimeter into the jungle with the Japs on the other side of that. We took on three squadrons of PTs—about 36 boats, and I had to take care of their crews as well as the crew of our ship. Our crew was involved in carpentry and mechanical duties, fixing up the PTs. The PTs patrolled the coastlines away from the beachheads to keep the Japs from moving troops by sea.

When we were on the ship at a place like Finchhaven, we didn't see much war. We occasionally went ashore and talked to some of the soldiers coming back from duty out on the perimeter. They would tell us stories about Japs trying to surrender because they were starving out there and couldn't be resupplied. However, this was an unusual occurrence for the Japanese warriors; they were brought up not to surrender.

From Finchhaven we moved to Hollandia, following MacArthur's path along the coast. We stayed at Hollandia for some time and then moved to Biack, an island off the northwest coast of New Guinea. It was to be the jump-off place for the invasion of the Philippines. When we got there, it was completely controlled by American troops. There were some Japanese troops still in the jungle around the base, but they offered no real resistance. In fact, there were stories that every so often some of them would try to sneak in and get in the chow line. There were also stories that, at the night movies, occasionally two or three of them would sneak in and sit in the last row. But we never saw any action from them at all.

Biack was a most uncomfortable place. We were there at the end of September when the sun is right over the equator, and Biack is 1° south latitude, which is only 60 miles south of the equator. Quite a few of the crew, including me, broke out with heat rash such as I was used to seeing on babies. I found that we could go over to the beach, where sitting in the salt water and letting the waves break over us would help the heat rash considerably.

It didn't take us long to find out what the war was all about. We had not been anchored more than three or four hours when there was a major air attack by suicide planes. Fortunately, very near where we were anchored we had an airstrip—serviceable on land—and some fighter planes which, though not many, were active. A freighter that was anchored close to us was hit by a suicide plane. We could see the damage, the flames and the destruction of it very well from our ship. I remember thinking of the fact that men had lost their lives there and the families at home would be notified. This made us realize that the war was really on here, as far as we were concerned.

We began to know late in August that there were preparations for the landings in the Philippines and that the war would take on a different aspect for us at that stage.

The first invasion of the Philippines by MacArthur was October 9, 1944. We followed about two weeks later. We went up in a convoy with our PT boats—under their own power—going along with us. We carried 50,000 gallons of aviation fuel, high-grade gasoline and 16 torpedoes in torpedo racks in the center of the ship—so we were highly flammable as far as air attacks went. Just before we reached the Philippines, I was promoted to lieutenant.

We arrived at the beachhead at Leyte Gulf where the original landings were made in the Philippines, about ten days after the first landings. As we started up Leyte Gulf early one morning, general quarters sounded, and word was passed that a fairly sizable group of Japanese bombers seemed to be headed our way. We were in the outside row of the convoy, the last ship in the row. We had heard that the

Japanese had a way of taking on those particular positions in a convoy, so we began to think we were going to get our first real taste of war. However, none of the Japs showed up, and we went on up the Leyte Gulf and anchored just off the airstrip at Tacoma, which is at the very top of the gulf on the island of Leyte. At that time, the airstrip there was the only strip on Leyte and had about fifteen fighter planes and a few small twin-engine bombers.

We received a communiqué from MacArthur that he had complete control of the air over Leyte. In the next 24 hours, we counted 29 air raids, which some of us thought was not an indication of complete control. We had almost constant air raids for the next several weeks, mostly by suicide planes, and several close calls—planes that were shot down as they dived to hit us and fell into the water close to us.

Thanksgiving was a memorable day. The refrigerated navy supply ships had brought in turkeys, and we were having a big holiday dinner. We received food just like we were at home. The poor old Army was over on the shore eating Spam. The captains and the officers of all the PT boats came on board for the meal. The action started at about one o'clock. We had four air raids—one after the other—with suicide bombers, and it took us two and one-half hours to finish dinner because of jumping up to man the battle stations.

During November and December, we were very heartened by the arrival of Admiral Halsey's large fleet, which contained all of the big aircraft carriers that the Navy had. He came in and started up at Formosa—now Taiwan—and in about three days, he attacked every airfield from Formosa on down to below where we were in the Philippines.

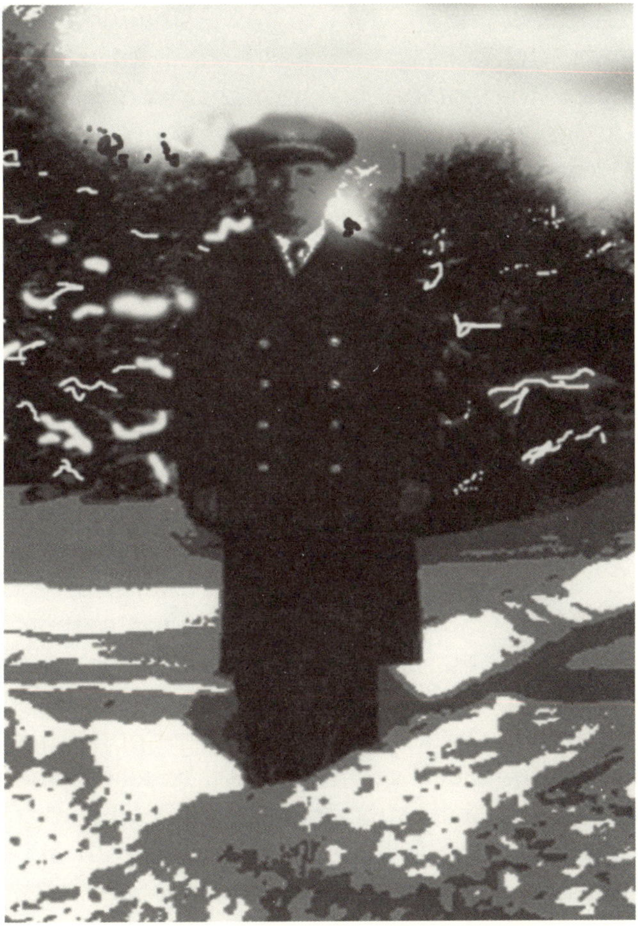

Lieutenant (jg) Lewis Standish Rathbun

In mid-December, we began to know through the usual "grapevine" that we were going to have significant action. We learned that there were preparations for MacArthur to land on Luzon to try to take Manila. There was to be an attack on Mindoro, which was a small island south of Manila. The goal was to build an airstrip for fighter coverage of the landings on Luzon that would position us to take Manila in mid-January. As the preparations went on, we knew we were going to have a big part in it. We heard among the higher-ups that there had been some question about whether to send our ship up there. As I've said, it was lightly defended, and there were thoughts that it couldn't possibly survive over a period of time in that area with the strong Japanese air attacks that were sure to come.

However, word came. We were going to Mindoro, and it would be a very hazardous journey.

This of course set everyone thinking, including myself. Over a period of days we had to face head-on the fact that we would be in extreme danger, and there was a possibility that we would be killed. During this time, I was rather surprised that in my thinking and emotions—not really praying but thinking about life and God—I seemed to reach an inner peace. I finally got to the point that I was resigned to the fact that I might well be killed, and I did not seem to be particularly afraid. I felt sorry that my family would be put through the sorrow of my death, should it come, and I was sorry that I would not see my baby who had been born in October. But I was more sorry for them than I was for myself.

We did get hit, and I narrowly escaped being killed. Things turned out for me but not for many of the others. Since then, I don't think I have really felt the degree of inner peace I found at that time.

In order to get to Mindoro, we had to go in passageways between several of the small islands in the Philippines and along the coast and pass a big island highly fortified by the Japs. There were many Japanese air fields that covered the route.

We had been getting Christmas presents from home most of December. The crew would usually open their presents when they arrived, but I decided to save mine for Christmas unless we left for Mindoro before Christmas, in which case I would open them before we left. We were able to have Christmas before departure and enjoyed a good turkey dinner. A Catholic priest in the chaplains' corps came aboard and held services for the Catholics and a service for the Protestants; I think everybody on the ship went to both services because we knew what was ahead of us.

We were the third convoy to start for Mindoro. We departed at about five o'clock at night on December 26, and this turned out to be as bad as we thought it would be. We left with thirty ships in the convoy just as dusk fell. The route was quite long, winding in and out of the islands, although it wasn't very far by air. Supposedly, we were going to get fighter cover from the Army Air Corps there at the base in Leyte. When dawn broke the next morning, there was no air cover. In the first hour and a half of daylight, we lost six ships out of the thirty, with constant air attacks by suicide planes. One of the casualties was an ammunition ship, a 10,000-ton liberty ship loaded with ammunition. It was the next ship ahead of us in convoy. It was about 600 yards from us when a suicide plane dove down the forward hold, exploding the whole ship. The explosion blew in a bulkhead on our ship. I had been in the wardroom with a patient. There was a tremendous crash, and our ship lurched to the side. I thought we'd been hit. I pushed open a hatch to see what the situation was. The

10,000-ton liberty ship had completely disappeared. There wasn't anything left of that ship; there wasn't even debris on the water. All that remained was a great puff of smoke. There was one survivor. He was picked up unconscious in the water about 1500 feet from our ship. One of the PTs rescued him.

One quiet afternoon I was standing out on deck, watching one of our destroyers out on our flank. It was a cloudy day, the clouds maybe at 1500 feet. All of a sudden, the warship made a very sharp turn and headed at full speed down the side of our convoy. As it got partway down the convoy, the forward, five-inch gun fired one shell. In a few seconds, pieces of plane came floating down out of the clouds. Despite the clouds, the radar had detected the enemy plane, and the gun had fired accordingly. We were eternally grateful for that marksmanship. After three nights and two days, we anchored at about three in the afternoon at Mindoro. The assault troops had been ashore for several days. They had established a beachhead, carved out a very rough airport with a runway for fighter planes, and established an Army hospital there.

Everyone on our ship was exhausted. Those who did not have duty went to their quarters. I went down to my state room that I shared with another officer and went to sleep. In about an hour, we were awakened by the General Quarters alarm and jumped up. I started out, simultaneously donning my life jacket and helmet. I had to go straight up a corridor to the ward room to set up the operating supplies. As I came to the door of my cabin, there were several line officers running up the corridor. I stepped back in my cabin to get out of their way because it was more important for them to get where they were going. Just after I had stepped back, there was a crash and explosion. We'd been hit by a suicide plane.

When I looked out in the corridor again, all those officers were piled up in front of my door, dead. Two suicide planes had come in at once. One of them hit a destroyer that was anchored very near us and did some severe damage. The one that hit us came in low over the water and dropped his bomb before he got to the ship. The bomb had skipped off of the water like a stone. Apparently, it was an armor-piercing bomb that would not explode on impact. Of course, as a PT tender, we were not heavily armored. The bomb was able to pass through the side of the ship into the center, right into the room where sixteen torpedoes were stacked. They were stored in slots formed by steel girders running up from floor to ceiling and then crossways at intervals.

Fortunately, instead of hitting a torpedo, the bomb hit one of the steel stanchions and went straight up through the overhead bulkhead into the boiler room and detonated up there. That exploded both boilers. In that room was one of the large damage-control parties. They had responded to the General Quarters alarm and were blown to bits. The boiler room was right ahead of the ward room to which I had been en route. It blew out that bulkhead. There were two officers in the ward room and they were both killed.

The attack started a fire. We had fifty thousand gallons of aviation fuel in the fore part of the ship that was in danger of going up, as well as the sixteen torpedoes. No one could predict whether they would go off or not. With no boilers, there was no power and thus no way of fighting the fire, so we were ordered to abandon ship. Some of the PTs that were around us came up, and the captains of the PTs said, "Give us your wounded."

We assisted getting the injured off. The landing craft that were nearby came out to us, but for safety concerns, didn't get too close. We had to jump off the ship and swim out to the rescue boats that took us ashore to the small PT base. Out of the crew of three hundred, forty-nine had been killed.

There was an army hospital at the air base where there was a newly-made airfield. The runway consisted of steel sheeting, rather than dirt or macadam. It was a rough ride, but the planes got on and off. I helped put the critically wounded and burned on the narrow-gauge train—ordinarily used to bring sugar cane in from the fields. I accompanied them in transport to the hospital. We tried to be as secretive as possible, but it was a moonlit night and the wood fire in the monstrous engine spewed a steady stream of huge sparks out the smokestack. But no bombs were dropped. I remember one officer I knew quite well whose foot was nearly blown off at the ankle and was attached by a little tag of skin. A thought crossed my mind, *At least he'll be going home and out of all this.*

Back at the PT base, when the fire burned down and it became obvious that the torpedoes were not going to detonate, nor the gasoline catch fire and explode, the anchor chain was cut. Some of the small boats pushed the Orestes into shore. The next day, we had to retrieve the bodies of those who had been killed—a most unpleasant task. A small military morgue had been made on a hill near the airport. The bodies were taken there, cataloged and buried.

Official naval inspectors arrived and went over the ship, which had been grounded. They thought it was worth repairing the engines. Because the engines were caput, they had to tow us back to Leyte with a Naval tug. On the earlier trip to Leyte, we had traveled amid constant air raids, but now, coming back to Leyte, there were no air raids to threaten a tug and a crippled ship. We weren't worth foolin' with.

At Leyte, after considerable repair work, a decision was made to take the Orestes back to Pearl Harbor for major construction, and it was determined that we could leave under our own power. I thought, *In a month's time, they could have built a new one in the United States.*

On January 29, we set off for the long journey—despite reservations—because of the orders from the powers that be. We started out with one engine, creeping along to Pearl Harbor. All the explosives had detonated in the middle of the ship and had gutted the essential workings. It didn't look like a very safe vessel. If I stood in the back of the ship and a sizable wave came along, I could see the ship bend in the middle. The sides would go up, and the middle would go down. It made a loud cracking noise. We wondered if we would one day wake up on half a ship.

Still there were no air raids because the enemy had no control of the air in those areas. Enemy submarines were still a risk, but most of their carriers had been demolished.

Our first stop was in Eniwetok—now Enewetak—which is an atoll in the middle of the Pacific where hydrogen bombs were later tested. It was a beautiful spot—a central island surrounded by a 15 to 20-mile circle of little islets created by a volcano. It was a wonderful place for ships to come in because there was a narrow inlet into this big bay that was easily defended against submarines. I could see the rocks—even sharks—on the bottom, 75 feet below, as clearly as if I were looking into my own bathtub.

An atoll consists of a group of small islands in a big circle. The circle was about fifteen miles in diameter. It formed a wonderful harbor inside, so big ships could come in. On the small islands around Eniwetok, various things had been set up. For example, there was an officers' club, serving rum and coke. A bartender would put ice in a glass and stand and pour rum from a bottle for a dime and then, while talking to us, would add a splash of coke. There was a special bar for those with a gold leaf—at least a rank of commander, the same as lieutenant colonel in the Army.

We were there to get more orders and to rest. During that time, Admiral Halsey's Task Force 58 came in and anchored. I will never forget that sight. There were twelve or fourteen of the biggest carriers and five or six big battleships, including the tremendous North Carolina and the Missouri. There were over fifty cruisers and seventy-five destroyers. They were the main force for the Pacific fleet. They were preparing to go in for the invasion of Okinawa because there had been heavy fighting in the efforts to capture it, since it had been heavily defended by the Japanese. The Navy wanted to build an airbase there. By that time, the Philippines had been pretty well secured. Halsey was one of the finest combat admirals. His force would come down in a sweep and wipe out all the Japanese airbases en route. When we heard he was on one of his sorties, we knew we would have three to four days of no Kamikazes. He had destroyed all the planes. Then they would resupply them from Japan, and the "fun" would began again.

There were several atolls in the Marshall Islands. I had found out that there was a physician from my little home town of Phelps on one of the other atolls. The Navy had a machine shop set up there that repaired landing crafts. So one afternoon, I got my crew to take me over with one of the boats from the ship. After I spent the afternoon with the doctor, he wanted me to stay for dinner and watch a movie. He said his people would take me back to my ship.

Eniwetok was about seventy-five miles from Palau, which was an island held by the Japs. It had an air strip on it. Our forces bombed it regularly, so it was thought to have absolutely no airplanes on it that were serviceable, and nobody paid much attention to it. We were watching the movie outdoors on the coral that night. All of a sudden, a loudspeaker came on. "Flash red! Flash red! All Army personnel, man your battle stations!"

Having been through the recent attack on our ship, I was a bit alert and said to my friend, "Shouldn't we be going somewhere?"

He said, "Oh no, that's just an Army thing. They call an alert every time a barrel floats by out there. There is nothing out here."

Just about the time he finished saying it, from the carrier Franklin, which was anchored where we could see it, there was this tremendous explosion. Flames shot way up into the air off the flight deck. The loudspeaker blared again. "Flash Red, Flash Red! This is not drill! This is not a drill!"

Then we heard a plane coming near us, and to me, it didn't sound like one of ours. I had heard enough Jap planes, so I said to the guys around me, "Duck and get under something!"

We were all flat on the coral, trying to scoop out a place with our bare hands. The plane crashed into the island about two hundred to three hundred yards from us. Later, when they examined the wreckage, they found two pilots in it. My thought was, Didn't that plane have two pilots in it? Why they would send two pilots on a suicide mission, I don't know. None of the Americans was hurt, but an inspection of the wreckage showed it was made up of parts of American planes. What they had done, apparently, was cannibalize some planes that had been shot down over Palau and built three to four planes. One of them had hit the carrier out there and did a lot of damage but didn't sink it. We figured he dove into the island because he probably took it for a carrier at night. It was the length of a carrier.

We left there and went on to Pearl Harbor. We finally arrived sometime in April. At Pearl, the Orestes was supposed to be repaired structurally; there was much more work needed. But before the repair crew got to our task, they had to turn their attention to two of Halsey's big carriers that had been severely damaged in the Okinawa invasion. Halsey's force had been to Okinawa, and from there his damaged ships reached Pearl at 30 knots per hour in the time it took our damaged ship to get there from Eniwetok, covering the distance at only 8 knots per hour. They came in just after we got there. It was much more important to get them going, so they just put us aside and started working on them night and day to get them back into service. They eventually decided to send the Orestes back to California to be worked on. There were no dissenting votes from the crew. In fact, we were mighty happy about that.

The end of October, 1944, when we were in the Philippines, I began to look for word of our first child, who was due at the end of October. The Red Cross sent all the servicemen telegrams, which might or might not be delivered any time soon, and, of course, the general mail, which eventually caught up with us. I think it was about the sixth or seventh of November when I received a letter that said a baby girl had been born on October 31 and everything was fine. In the midst of all the air raids and suicide planes, I had hoped through October that I would live to find out who the baby was, and then I began to hope that I would see a picture of her, which I did in late December. She was given the name Alexandra—"Lexie."

It took us eight or nine more days to get to California. We went into Long Beach Naval Station. They gave half the ship's crew leave at a time. I had to stay there for the first two weeks and then got leave, went home and saw

Betty and my daughter Lexie. They were with my folks in Phelps. I was overjoyed to see my daughter, my wife and my family.

The enlisted men got train tickets to their destinations. I was given an airplane ticket on a DC3 commercial flight. I got into Rochester after twenty-four hours out of Los Angeles—with many stops.

My family knew our ship had been hit and that there had been deaths. We were not allowed to write who had been killed, but we learned ways to get around it without violating the requirement. Betty had been in Norfolk at the time with the officer's wives. I had written regularly. There were seventeen officers, a lot of whom Betty knew. I would name the ones still alive and state that they "send their regard to you." She noted the names of the people missing from the letter and, on her own, figured out what had happened. I might say, "It probably would be a good idea not to write to . . . until you hear from her."

We also could not identify our location in our letters. So when my brother wrote and said he knew that Goff was up at Landia, New Guinea, I wrote back, "Last I heard, Goff was in Buffalo, New York." Dick would then know to calculate the distance from Buffalo to Phelps and transpose it to the distance I was east of Goff's location. My mother wrote once complaining that there was never any news except whether the ice-cream maker was working. The censors would surely have had no part of the detail she wanted.

The townspeople themselves were already used to seeing soldiers return with no arm or no leg. The church held a dinner for three or four of us who returned home. There was a dance at the school where I renewed some old acquaintances.

While I was in Phelps, my orders came through transferring me off our PT tender, the Orestes, and onto the Naval Air Station in Atlanta, Georgia. I was glad to get the new assignment because I didn't relish going back out in the Pacific. It would be more to my liking because at least I could feel I knew what I was doing—what I had been trained to do.

We all knew that we were going to have to land on Japan in order to terminate the war. The plans were well underway for such landings. Of course, we knew nothing of the atom bomb at that stage of the game. Those of us who had seen the ferocity with which the Japanese fought, even hand-to-hand, and their willingness to die for the emperor, were certain that any attempt to take Japan itself, no matter how decimated the armed forces of Japan were, would be an extremely bloody affair.

I had to fly back to Long Beach to the ship to get my official orders, sign out and get what clothes were left. I took the train back to Phelps where I still had a few days' leave. Jeannette MacDonald, the actress, had a compartment on the same train. Then I took my car, an old Chrysler, which had been up on blocks the whole time I was gone, and drove to Atlanta. Betty and Lexie stayed with my folks because I didn't yet have a place to stay in Atlanta.

When I got to the Naval Air Station, I started looking for a place so that they could join me. It took me about two weeks. It was very difficult because Atlanta was bursting at the seams with Army personnel and people working in factories.

The Naval Air Station in Atlanta was a subsidiary of the big Pensacola Naval Air Station where pilots were trained. The base had 2,000 Waves on it, and I was the only obstetrician/gynecologist. I also had the responsibility for all of the naval dependents who lived in the area of Atlanta.

The Navy took care—medically speaking—of the families of anyone who was in the Navy. So in addition to taking care of the Waves, I was doing pediatrics and general medicine. We also were assigned to take night duty at the infirmary in rotation.

It was a busy life with only eight or ten doctors there. We had a good surgeon and a good internist. All physicians were reserve officers except the captain, who was the senior medical officer there. The regular Navy medical officers, who had gone up in the ranks as high as captain, had been in the Navy all through the '20s and '30s and really hadn't practiced much medicine. They left the actual clinical work mostly to the reservists. We did all of the obstetrics and quite a bit of surgery in addition to managing a variety of illnesses. I had to treat everything from back aches to fevers.

We had registered nurses who were also Navy personnel. We had scrub nurses who were reserve enlisted men who had been trained in operating room work. One scrub nurse had been a barn painter up in Indiana. He had been well trained and was an excellent nurse in the operating room. Before I came, he had gained quite a bit of experience. He was as good as anybody there, helping me with hysterectomies and other gynecologic surgical procedures. I always wondered what kind of tales he would later tell his fellow painters out in the farmland of Indiana.

The senior medical officer—a regular naval officer of many years—knew almost no clinical medicine. He was good, I guess, at shuffling papers. There was going to be a Commandant's Inspection of the infirmary, and we had prepared for it for several days. Everything had to be spit and polish and just so. It was going to start at nine o'clock on Saturday morning when the commandant would arrive. He would go over the entire infirmary with the senior medical officer. The captain was in a tizzy about everything going right.

About an hour before the inspection started, a woman was admitted in labor. I thought she needed a cesarean section, and I planned to do one on her. Actually, there was no great rush about it, but I thought, Well, let's just see what happens to the day's plans when I add this to the mix. I went to the senior medical officer and said, "I've got a woman who just came in who needs a cesarean, and I plan to go ahead and do it."

He answered, "Well, you can't do that. We've got this inspection. It will foul up the operating room."

I said, "Well, she needs it, and she ought to have it, and I think I'm going to have to go on and do it." After receiving a great remonstrance that was just short of being ordered to cancel the plan, I said, "Okay, I won't do it, but I'll write in the record that it ought to be done now."

He said, "Well, if you've got to . . . well . . . go ahead."

So I started the cesarean just as the captain and the commandant stuck their heads in the door. The captain said, "I'm so sorry, Commander, Dr. Rathbun thinks he has to do this cesarean right now. I'm so sorry we are in the middle of this."

The commandant said, "That's what the operating room is for, isn't it?" Then he said, "Dr. Rathbun, would you mind if I came in and watched?"

I said, "Oh, that would be fine." We got him a gown, cap and mask. He came in, watched the operation and stayed and talked about how wonderful it was and how everything had gone so well. He never did finish the inspection. It was kind of funny to see the various reactions from the old navy captain. When the commander started praising us, he bustled up ready to take all the credit.

As July progressed, we were sure that the United States was going to win the war very handily. But "very handily" was likely to include an invasion of Japan. Army planners predicted as many as a million or more casualties, and I figured we were likely to be among them. MacArthur loved PTs, so we assumed we would be anchored like sitting ducks off Japan's coast. They were drawing up plans. Jerry, my fraternity brother when we were in Hamilton, said, "I hope I'll get pushed into some actual fighting because I've been sitting here in this office at the army base in Honolulu the whole war."

I said, "It's nothing to want to get into if you don't have to."

Then the news of the atom bomb came, and it looked for sure as though the war would be over in a very few days.

We heard it at the base before it came over the public radio. Right off the bat, it occurred to me that the bomb could be a serious thing for civilization in general. I remember going home with the news. I remember telling Betty that there was a bomb and it had done so much damage. I said, "This will end the war, but we may regret that such a bomb was ever developed." I was with my family when the word came over the radio first. I remember picking up Lexie and holding her and saying, "They're not going to be shooting at your father anymore."

It wasn't much of a problem taking care of the Waves. They had the regular GYN problems that women 18 to 40 have. Their gynecologic care made up most of the practice as well as delivering babies for both the Waves and the dependents. Many of the dependents' husbands were not at the base. They could be anywhere in the world. The wife of one submarine captain was about seven months pregnant as the war ended. Her husband's submarine was the last one sunk just before the armistice. When she got the news she went into labor at seven months.

If I found in an examination that a Wave was pregnant, I sent a letter up the chain of command to the senior medical officer and up to the commandant. She received an honorable discharge and could go home with nothing further being done. However, the girls—as women were often called then—caught on to the fact that if the pregnancy wasn't discovered until very late, and they could go into labor before they were discharged, they could have the baby there, arrange for the baby to be adopted and then be discharged and go home. Therefore, they tried to put off being discovered with the pregnancy for as long as possible. One Saturday noon, a young woman appeared in my office in fairly active labor. The night before, she had played third base on a women's baseball team in a big exposition game. No one in any chain of command knew that she was pregnant during that entire game. She delivered an eight-pound baby about three hours after arrival.

We had walk-in office hours, but we had no waiting room; the people sat in chairs along the wall in the hallway. One day a woman from Atlanta came into my office. The first thing she said to me was, "I am very surprised that you would take Negro patients here."

This took me by surprise. "Well, as far as I know, that woman's husband is in the Navy just the same as yours."

A strange, reflective look came over her face. After a pause, she said, "Well, I suppose that's so." This was the first time I had seen people who seemed to feel that blacks were not like whites.

In the process of taking care of dependents, I ran into things that were not covered in obstetrics-gynecology training. The nonmilitary doctors in Atlanta were very good about helping me out with cases when I didn't feel adequate, like the care of premature babies. I tried not to call on them any more than I could help because they were frantically busy. So many doctors had left Atlanta for the service that those remaining were working tremendously long hours. Nevertheless, the few that I knew never refused to come out for a consultation on a hospitalized patient.

I remember a woman with severe hypertension who was delivering a very premature baby. I called a pediatrician and said, "We have no facilities for the baby, and with her condition, she'll never be able to have another." He put the baby in a little satchel like a suitcase—barely larger than a doctor's bag—and took it into the premature nursery in Atlanta.

In the Spring of 1946, after a little over two and one-half years, I was dismissed, having served the required time, and was very glad to be out of the service. I was proud to have served my country, but I had also seen the negative side of war. Our planes would go over an area where the Japanese had been pushed back and were isolated without food and would drop leaflets with Japanese writing that said, "If you want food, come out of the woods naked" (to avoid the risk of hand grenades hidden in the clothing). I heard soldiers talk about the expressions on their faces when they emerged, naked, following instructions, holding the flyer, and then were shot point-blank. No prisoners were to be taken because a wounded Japanese soldier would be lying there, and a corpsman would try to help him. The fallen man would reach under his shirt and kill both of them. No medical officers carried a side arm until this started happening. However, they understood the delicate balance between compassion and mortal jeopardy.

But the Japanese did much the same thing. If one of our PTs had to be abandoned on an enemy shoreline, the enemy would come out on board and just decapitate them all. I heard that after peace documents were signed, Japanese guards running prisons, for example with pilots shot down, were so upset they took ten or twelve prisoners out and decapitated them.

Early in the winter of 1946, it became obvious that I would be eligible for discharge soon—probably early May or late April—and my thoughts turned to what I was going to do then. There was some pressure from regular Navy people to stay in the Navy, but I didn't want to do that. Having one child and another on the way, I had to begin to figure out how to make a living.

During the war, people I knew in obstetrics/gynecology in both Rochester and Boston had indicated that they would like to have me come there, but as the end of the war approached, and people began to get out of the medical corps and come back to where they had been, the attitude of the men who had stayed home during the war changed. They began to say there were too many men coming back to give me a place in their private practice.

About the time I was getting out of the service, doctors were beginning to form groups of physicians, usually with several different specialties in a group. There were more of these in the Midwest than anywhere else. I contacted individuals at a service in Chicago that I learned about from the Journal of the American Medical Association (JAMA). They advertised that they placed physicians in these groups. They sent me the names of several that wanted an obstetrician/gynecologist.

In mid April, I took Betty back up to Phelps to stay with my family. She was due to deliver by the end of May. I had hoped I would be out of the Navy before then. I didn't want her to stay in Atlanta and deliver down there because I didn't know how I could take care of her. I flew her and our first child, Lexie, from Atlanta back up to Rochester. I went back to the base and stayed there until I was discharged. Then I drove up to the Midwest and looked at several of the clinics who wanted an obstetrician, and all of them offered me jobs. I picked the one in Rockford, Illinois, and returned to Phelps in time to be present when my second daughter, Linda, was born.

We rented a house in Phelps, and after Betty and the two girls got settled in, I took several days in Boston to see what medical news had developed while I had been in the Navy. In Boston, I heard that one of the men I admired the most in Ob/Gyn had expressed an interest sometime before that in taking me on. I had never learned about this because of my war service and so, of course, I hadn't contacted him. As soon as I learned of it, I got in touch with him immediately, but he had already hired someone else. Disappointed, I went on to Chicago to take the Illinois State Boards. I would loved to have joined him. He was the only one on the staff at Lying-In who had the courage to stand up to Dr. Irving. The Professor would make a certain statement in an authoritative manner. Dr. Smith would say, "Now, wait a minute . . ." when the others would say, "Yes, sir . . ."

4

MEDICAL PRACTICE

One of the most interesting cases I remember involved what is called placental abruption. The placenta suddenly separates from the uterine wall. The resulting hemorrhage can be extremely heavy.

I was called by a Canton family practitioner to come right to the hospital, where he had a patient four-and-one-half months pregnant and bleeding heavily. By the time I got there, I was able to extract the pre-viable baby as a breech and get the placenta out. The bleeding stopped, and the patient recovered well.

The next time I saw her, she was bleeding at about seven months with a new pregnancy. Her doctor put her into an ambulance and sent her to Asheville. She had another placental separation and was able to deliver from below. The baby died because it was too premature.

A year or two later, he again sent the patient, this time with a more advanced separation, and the whole process happened quicker. The baby was dead by the time she arrived at the hospital. She lost so much blood before and after delivery, she eventually required eleven transfusions in order to bring her blood count up to normal.

When she got pregnant again, he asked me if I would do her prenatal care. I had warned her of the very early symptoms of a placental abruption. When she was about eight months pregnant, she called and said she had a severe backache, one of the warning signs. I told her to get to the hospital as fast as she could. While she was en route, I rallied a team for a cesarean section set up. They were ready to go when she got in the emergency room, and we did a very rapid operative delivery. At that time, she was not bleeding; she had only a severe backache. By the time we got into the abdomen, we could see the blood streaks flaring out through the uterine muscle. I was extremely happy for this woman to get a live baby because she had gone through so much trying to do so.

ROCKFORD, ILLINOIS

We moved out to Rockford about the first of July, 1946. Fifteen years after graduation from high school, I started my medical practice.

In medical school and in residency, no one had told us how to start a practice. I thought it would be a very slow process. I had the idea that I would need to go into a place and become known by joining clubs and other social organizations. It turned out that it was actually much easier than I thought. There were—in any city, always—individuals who didn't care for the work of the specialist there and were ready to try a new doctor. In addition, there were doctors who would send patients to new people just as a way of helping them get started.

The general quality of medicine in the Rockford area at that time was not what I was used to. We really didn't care for Rockford after spending an extremely hot summer and an extremely cold winter, and I was not terribly happy with the way I was having to practice. The following year, I got an offer to join a clinic in Asheville, North Carolina. I had heard while I was in Atlanta what a wonderful place Asheville was in which to live—up in the mountains of the western part of the state. I applied for the job and received what I considered to be a very good offer. We moved to Asheville, and I took the position of head of Ob/Gyn at the Norburn Clinic.

ASHEVILLE, NORTH CAROLINA

In September 1947, we moved to Asheville. At the time we moved, we had the two children, and Betty was pregnant again. She delivered our third daughter, Laurel, in November. Our three children were each a year and a half apart. You might wonder if I delivered my daughters. I was overseas when my first daughter was delivered, so it wasn't even an option. But I did not deliver the other two. In those days fathers weren't even in the delivery room—that was unheard of. But in deference to my medical status, I was able to sit in the doctors' dressing room instead of the general waiting room.

Group Practice

Three people had started the Norburn Clinic—two were brothers in their mid-50s who had practiced in Asheville for years. One of the brothers was a surgeon and the other one did various things such as some nose-and-throat medicine and some urology. Neither of them were specialty-trained, but the surgeon had a little extra medical education and was a pretty good technician. The third was a general practitioner whose father was the CEO of Champion Paper Company.

They had added a good internist from Duke and a highly-trained young surgeon who came from Cincinnati, from a program turning out excellent operating physicians. After I came as head of Ob/Gyn, we added a man who had been in the Navy and had some Ob/Gyn training at Great Lakes. He was not yet qualified by the boards when he came to work with me. We also added a second general practitioner, another excellent internist from Johns Hopkins and a pathologist. One of the men from the city did our radiology and the small amount of radiation therapy that was performed.

We had our own hospital. Norburn Clinic had taken over a teacher's college—Asheville Normal School. The main, large brick building acted as a 55 – 65 bed hospital. We had a good general manager and good equipment.

Many of our patients came from outlying areas. We had a big practice from Canton and Waynesville where Champion Paper Company conducted a very large and prosperous business. Also, I developed quite a practice from Marion and Black Mountain—nearby small towns.

We had, of course, patients from Asheville. A clinic like this starting up did not sit very favorably with doctors in town. The idea of the people who started the clinic—the two brothers and the family practitioner—was to build a second Mayo Clinic. They made a point of adding well-trained people who practiced excellent medicine. Some of the local doctors were not happy about a group of well-trained people coming in and diluting the practices that they had. We got little support from them. In fact, there was considerable antagonism in the early days.

Early in my time in Asheville, in fact, in the first month or two, I was surprised to see the level of some aspects of practice in the community. I put my energy into seeking changes and, to a degree, found a responsive community. For instance, there was no prenatal clinic for any indigent patients as recently as sixty years ago. I went down to the county health department and offered to run a prenatal clinic if I were to be given a place to run it and some nurses to help me. The health officer was overjoyed at this, and we started a prenatal clinic for those who couldn't afford private care.

Most of the people who came to the clinic were "colored"—the term used at that time for Afro-American individuals. There were four colored midwives working in town, and they asked me to instruct them. This was early in my career, and I had little experience with the level of training of colored nurses or midwives. In my first lecture, I assumed that these caregivers had been to some sort of a school for midwives and had been properly trained. I hadn't proceeded five minutes in the lecture when the public health nurse who was there stopped me and said that I had to use different language so that they would understand. For example, they didn't know what I was talking about when I referred to the vagina and the rectum. I quickly learned that I was to refer to the "front passage" and the "back passage." The need to use a variety of other very common terms surprised me greatly and let me know immediately what the situation had been as far as obstetrics for the poor in Asheville.

I told the midwives to call me if they ever got in trouble with a home delivery and I'd come out and try to help them. This did not happen often, but occasionally, I'd go out.

I remember one morning in the summer when one of the midwives called me and said that she had a patient bleeding a lot more than she should. "Would you please come up and help me?" It was about 5:30 in the morning.

When I arrived in the area, I thought I was near the place, but I couldn't find it. Most of the houses didn't have numbers on them. I got as close as I could to where I thought I should be, got out of the car, went up to a house and knocked on the door. I knocked and knocked but nobody came. Finally, I saw a curtain open so that I knew somebody was there, and finally, the door opened a crack. I could see there was a woman inside. "I am Dr. Rathbun," I said. "Mary Mosley, the midwife, called me and said a patient was delivering and was bleeding way too much and would I come up and help her."

She said, "Oh, that must be Mrs. Brown who lives right next door."

There was a black hospital in Asheville that left a great deal to be desired. The equipment was outdated, and the nursing was limited. I couldn't always depend on notations in the chart. I remember one patient I had who had preeclampsia, the condition of high blood pressure, protein in the urine and swelling toward the end of pregnancy. I admitted her and left orders for her to have her blood pressure taken every four hours and I would come twice a day and check her blood pressure. The whole time she was in there, her blood pressure was always 138/72 on the charts. I would take it and determine that, of course, it varied, albeit in the normal range. I continued to watch with great interest as the blood pressure never changed by one millimeter the whole time she was in the hospital . . . according to the notations in the record.

Most of the older obstetricians didn't take colored patients, and I guess for a while, I was the only one that did. My office, I am sorry to say, did tend to give them appointments late in the day. We certainly didn't charge them very much. Most of them were living on a very low income and just couldn't afford anything.

One of the black doctors used me a great deal for consultation. He was older than I and was a stickler for correct etiquette in contrast to most of the white doctors.

If he asked me to come out to the house to see a patient, he would always meet me there and would be scrupulously on time. He insisted, no matter how poverty-stricken the family looked, that I charge them something. His idea was that they had to assume responsibility, and therefore they must pay something, even if a small amount.

I remember going out late one week to see a colored minister's wife. As usual, the doctor met me there. We decided what should be done. As I left, the minister asked me what he owed me, and I had a hard time asking anything, but I said $2, and he said, "I'll pay you on Wednesday, depending on what the collection is on Sunday."

All physicians in the community had to take their black patients to the colored hospital because the other hospitals did not admit them. The black doctors initially only worked at the colored hospital and later were given staff positions at the other hospitals.

One case at the colored hospital stands out in my mind. It was a great tragedy. The same doctor who used me in consultation called me one night about 6:30 and said he had a patient at term who was bleeding very heavily, but there was no hurry going down to see her because he had packed her with gauze to stop the bleeding. In most cases, this was the worst thing a physician could do. I went down as quickly as I could and found this woman bleeding through the packing in her vagina and quickly determined that she had a placenta previa. In such a case, the placenta grows down over the cervical opening, and as the cervix opens during labor it allows the placenta with all its large vessels to bleed very heavily.

The patient was already going into shock, and we had no blood bank. I immediately called for the family to bring in relatives to be crossmatched and then found that we had no facility to perform that procedure in the hospital.

We had to send all the relatives up to a laboratory in town to get crossmatched. In the meantime, I had ordered the operating room to be set up for an emergency cesarean.

The operating room was on the second floor. This woman weighed about 200 pounds and there was no elevator. She had to be carried up the stairs, and there was nobody there strong enough to do it. We had to call a black funeral home to get some men to come over and carry her to the operating room. By that time, I had sent for my usual assistant and a scrub nurse from the other hospital, and we got ready to do the section as fast as we could get the blood. Finally, we got a report that there was a match donor.

We had no professional anesthetist. Dr. Holt was going to give her drop ether. As the patient was going under, she got somewhat agitated and started yelling, "Goddamn!" at the top of her lungs.

Dr. Holt, as he was sitting there pouring ether, kept saying, "Lady, you might better be praying than swearing." By this time, she was in desperate condition because of all the bleeding and the inability to replace blood in a timely way. We got the baby out, but sadly, it was dead, apparently from lack of oxygen caused by the lack of blood supply. The uterus failed to contract because the patient was so far gone. In order to stop the bleeding, I took the uterus out as quickly as possible and then, just as we were closing her up, she died. I never will forget going out and starting down the stairs, and at the bottom of the stairs was this man with two little children, not more than 5 or 6 years old, looking up with fearful eyes. I had to tell them that their mother, his wife, was dead.

The government eventually required that the hospitals admit black patients and not segregate them. At St. Josephs, it was announced that blacks were going to eat in the regular dining room. There was no opposition for two weeks. Two or three sat at each table. They had intentionally spread out. But after a couple of weeks, they were back in their own dining room where they could comfortably carry on their own conversations. They had re-segregated themselves.

There was a time that Mission Hospital would take blacks and St. Josephs would if they had to. A black patient who had been a good worker at St. Josephs for years had a gynecology problem, and I sent her to the admissions office. The supervisor called me and said, "We would like her admitted to Mission."

I said, "This woman has worked hard for you for years, and she naturally wants to be there. I want her there. I'm not admitting her to Mission." When I arrived they had her in a private room. They did keep her.

I had a patient from Waynesville whose husband was a powerful Democrat in the area. When the hospitals had just begun to take black patients, she was admitted for surgery. He came on the telephone line in a very brusque manner. "My wife has just been put in a two-bed room with a black! Call the hospital and get that changed immediately!"

I responded, "I'm sure you voted for Johnson and I did not. Why don't you call him and get the rules changed?"

Apparently another tactic was used, because when I returned that night, she had been placed in a room with another white woman.

Asheville had some good cultural opportunities, such as a lecture series during the winter, but nothing like the city has now with the Asheville Community Theater, the Asheville Symphony, the very fine Art Museum, the Mineral Museum, community concerts and many other events.

We developed an interesting social life in Asheville. There wasn't a lot of time for it, as far as I was concerned, but we joined the Newcomer's Club. There were a lot of young people coming into Asheville after the war; we met some very interesting couples about our own ages and formed some lasting friendships. Also, we enjoyed good relationships with the younger doctors and their wives who had joined the clinic. We didn't have much social life with the other doctors in the community.

The Buncombe County Medical Society had monthly meetings, and at each meeting some doctor gave a scientific paper. The doctors from Norburn Clinic were asked to give quite a few of these papers. At the end of the year, there was an award given for the best paper, and for several years in a row, one or another of the doctors from Norburn got this award.

We had a large referral practice from family practitioners in Madison, Haywood and McDowell Counties and some from Henderson County and Yancey County. Some of these patients had been neglected and were very challenging. Some of the cancer patients' problems were especially complex and offered an interest we might not have gained in a general city practice somewhere else. When I would meet friends of mine from Boston at medical meetings, and we would discuss eclampsia and other problems of pregnancy that were very difficult, I would say, "I have had five or six patients sent to me with those problems in the last few months or the last year."

They would say, "Gosh, we've only seen three." It made for an interesting—but not lucrative—practice.

I had good relationships with several of the doctors in surrounding counties, and we became fast friends for life. They were very, very busy, and a lot of them did good work, but there were other doctors out there who didn't do very good work. With some, I knew I couldn't depend on their diagnoses. There were a couple of doctors way out in the mountains that I'm sure were drinking much too much "mountain dew," from the way they acted.

I soon learned which doctors I could trust regarding what was going on with patients. I used to marvel, and still do, at three or four of the doctors out in the mountains who had to cope with all sorts of diseases and problems and who were very good diagnosticians. They were outstanding people and did a tremendous amount of work. They were frequently up all night. One doctor from Madison County was extremely busy. When he got exhausted, he would go to the Battery Park Hotel and take a room and just stay there for two or three days, sleeping and resting.

Most of the doctors from the Canton area were quite good. There was no well-trained surgeon but most did some surgery. There was one doctor who took out almost everybody's appendix, it seemed. Others of them were not extremely skilled but didn't try to exceed their capabilities. They would send us the complicated cases.

One of the men who was the busiest and who did a great deal of surgery—and I think did it quite well, although he wasn't formally trained—used to call me, and I soon learned what was coming when he called. He would say he had this elderly patient he just wanted the very best for, so he was going to send her over to me. She would have a fibroid uterus—a womb with benign tumors that sometimes grow and cause troublesome bleeding. I knew that he was removing fibroid tumors almost every day, so I soon learned to sit and wait for the end of the conversation, because after that he would say something like, "By the way she has a blood pressure of 240 and is a bad diabetic and has some heart trouble." I knew that if he was going to refer me someone, it was going to be a very challenging patient, but I enjoyed my relationship with him and was glad that he did not try to take on those difficult cases.

There was a great deal of cancer of the cervix at the time. It was at the very beginning of the use of Pap smears to pick up the disease in an early and treatable stage. Very few doctors were doing the screening tests in Asheville, and women were not coming for early signs, such as abnormal bleeding. So a lot of the cancer of the cervix that I saw was very far advanced.

Treatment for cancer of the cervix was then, as it largely is to this day, radiation—X-ray therapy to the pelvic area and radium directly applied in the cervix. Two well-trained radiologists in town had a therapy machine, but the early equipment was far short of the precision of modern ones.

The therapy could cause quite a bit of trouble in itself. There was no radium available in the community, so the radiologists were just giving X-ray therapy, which was not adequate. There was some radium down at Rutherfordton. A wealthy industrialist in Marion had gone to Memorial Hospital, a cancer hospital in New York, and received radium therapy for his cancer of the bladder. He had been cured, so he bought a large amount of radium and brought it to a surgeon in Rutherfordton who had absolutely no training in how to use it. Many Asheville women with cancer of the cervix had gone down there for radium therapy and had been treated very badly. As a consequence, we saw a great many vaginal fistulas. In the typical case, the urinary bladder had been burned with radium so much that there was a hole from the bladder into the vagina. These were very difficult to repair. Some of them were impossible to repair. Most of the women had such far-advanced cancer that they didn't live very long anyway.

I called the physician in Rutherfordton and explained my concerns. I said to him, "You are putting radium in the cervix, but what are you doing for the possibility of spread to the surrounding tissues?"

He said, "Oh, I just lay a little radium on the skin creases of the groin."

I cringed. This would destroy the skin in that area without penetrating even close to the site of the tumor.

In the very early 1950s, I was taking care of the wife of the dean of a university in the mountains. She asked me if I would see her housekeeper. The housekeeper was about 38 years old and had been bleeding for a long time. She had a very far-advanced cancer of the cervix. I knew I couldn't cure her, but I could stop the bleeding with radiation and radium.

By that time the Asheville radiologists had radium and could use it very effectively. I made an appointment for her to start her radiation. She went back to her rural community and didn't keep the appointment. I called her employer, my patient who referred her, and told her, "You've got to get that woman back down here so we can give her some treatment for the bleeding."

"Well, she won't come," she said. "It was the first time in her life she had ever been to Asheville, and it scared her so much that she just refused to come back."

She didn't live very long past that, but we could have made her more comfortable with the therapy. I was amazed that anyone that age had never previously been to Asheville, only 60 – 70 miles away, and that when she did come, it scared her so much. It's hard to think of Asheville as a scary place . . . but to a woman who never left the hill country . . . I can understand.

Faith healers came to town. I remember one charismatic fellow who set up a tent on the outskirts of Asheville and started having meetings. People went in droves. The community physicians had a terrible time after that. He convinced people that diabetics could stop taking insulin—all they had to do was have faith. Three patients of mine who had cancer of the cervix and were under radiation treatment stopped the therapy. I hit on a way of getting them back.

"The Lord is going to cure me," a patient would say.

I would respond, "The Lord has given us radiation therapy, and that is the way he is going to cure you." Fortunately, the majority went back to treatment. This was a real problem with a lot of people. Some of them went back to their churches, didn't take any therapy and instead, would be prayed over, but most of them would take both the therapy and the prayer. That was fine. I had no problem with that.

I soon learned that I had to speak a new language to communicate with some of the people in the mountains. In remote mountain coves, people had very little contact with what we would call the "outside world," and they referred to lots of things in medicine by very different names. For instance, I had to learn that "opals" were ovaries and "ultras" were ulcers. Some of the talk was almost like I had learned in college studying Chaucer in early English literature. For instance, the women referred to their breasts as "breasties." Another thing stymied me the first few times I heard it. When I would ask the patient what the trouble was, she might say, "I'm not piert," or "I'm piert." It took me a little bit to realize that "piert" meant pert. They were referring to whether they felt well or not, or how badly they felt. They referred to being angry about something as being "ill." They would say, "Is somebody ill with you?"

The frequent intermarrying among distant family members within the isolated communities seemed to contribute to health problems at times.

When I moved to Asheville, there were, at first, not a lot of specialists in town, that is, well-trained and board-certified in their respective specialties. Four younger men, who were well trained in Ob/Gyn, all came to town at about the same time. While I went into the Norburn Clinic, the other three joined the established obstetricians in town. The men in town were physicians doing exclusively Ob/Gyn but who were not board-certified. The boards required two years of practice before a candidate took the examination. Two of us received our specialty certification in 1949, and the other two younger doctors soon followed suit. The same thing happened in other specialties. There were two board-certified surgeons in town, and one very well-qualified surgeon come to the Norburn Clinic the same time I did. Until that time, surgery was being done by general practitioners who had been doing surgery for years.

There was one well-trained internist who came to town sometime after I did. In the post-war years, the army separated many people from the service at a hospital near Asheville, and that brought an influx of well-trained people in various fields. When they came to be discharged into civilian life from the hospital, quite a few of them stayed on—well-trained internists and psychiatrists and several young lawyers. Some met young women in the community, married them and settled down. This created a group of younger medical people. Younger businessmen also came in, district sales people got out of the army and got jobs, and some people in the insurance business arrived. So we had a fairly large group of well-educated people descending on Asheville at essentially the same time.

Solo Practice

As time went on at Norburn Clinic, it became fairly obvious to some of us that the clinic could not maintain the standards that we had originally set for ourselves. Yet, the opposition of some of the city doctors kept us from expanding to the degree that we felt we should, so gradually the patient load was reduced. It finally became apparent that the clinic was not going to keep up. Several of us started our individual practices.

I enjoyed being on my own. I started in an office downtown and was amazed at how rapidly my practice grew. After I had been in private practice for a year or two, I shared the office with John Barber, a native of Asheville. He had done some intern work with us at Norburn and came back to town after he went back to Boston and Philadelphia to get specialty training in Ob/Gyn. I was happy with the arrangement. We didn't have a partnership, but we helped each other in surgery. This relationship lasted for years.

The practice continued to grow. There were not only patients from town, but also, patients from surrounding communities. I was building a very large consultation practice. The surgery was going well. The hospitals were quite well equipped. Obstetrics was very good at that time. Both St. Joe's and Mission Hospitals had obstetrics units. Some of the doctors did all their work at one and some at the other. As far as possible, patients could go to whichever hospital they wished. I did tell my patients if they went into labor and I had somebody in labor at one hospital, they would have to go there because I couldn't watch two people in two different hospitals at the same time.

I hadn't been in practice on my own very long before one of the doctors in town—who had a large Ob/Gyn practice and a wealthy clientele—asked me to come in with him. I declined, even though it would have probably been a very financially-rewarding situation. I was making enough to be happy and doing what I felt was best for my patients, so I stayed on my own and never regretted it.

After Norburn Clinic broke up, Mission Hospital took over the Norburn grounds and closed its hospital off Charlotte Street. An addition was put on Mission Hospital with a fairly large public subscription. Three hospitals went together: Mission, Norburn Hospital and Biltmore Hospital, which was a small hospital down in Biltmore Village. This was in the mid-1950s. There was a large capital campaign to enlarge the Norburn Hospital by building onto the front. When this was completed, there was room for the colored hospital to move patients in there. All of the medical facilities in Asheville were at that point used by both blacks and whites.

As my cancer practice increased, I became more and more interested in the psychological situation of cancer patients. In those days, cancer was viewed by the patient as a death sentence, even though we had a fair number of cures. Cancers of the cervix sometimes grew to a very large size because there weren't many Pap smears being done in those days, and women were not coming in to be checked.

In the early 1950s, a patient in her late 30s came in to my associates from out in the mountains with a very far advanced cancer of the cervix. She was bleeding heavily, and the cancer was very large, filling half of the vagina. There was no question that she could not be cured with radiation or radium, which was of relatively good quality by that time. However, it could be used to stop the bleeding.

Hopefully, she would get better and have a better life for a time. She was given the radiation, and the tumor shrunk down but did not completely disappear. About six months after the completion of the therapy, it started to grow again. When I saw her in consultation with my partner, the tumor had grown, as far as we could tell, all the way to the pelvic sidewalls and was filling the upper vagina and the pelvis. I rebiopsied the tumor. All biopsies came back positive. I told her that there was nothing more that could be done. We couldn't even do a palliative operation to remove the bulk of the tumor because it was attached to the pelvic sidewalls.

She listened very politely and then got up and said, "I believe I'll let Jesus cure me."

We said, "Fine." She left the office.

Two and one-half years later she came back into the office wanting a certificate for her church that she was cured. We examined her, and she didn't have any sign of cancer anywhere. We followed her for ten years after that, and she never developed any recurrence of the cancer. This was astounding—something that I never forgot. This case led me to watch the literature. Publications on the subject began in the 1960s. The experimental literature showed that mental attitude did have something to do with how people got along with cancer and probably other serious diseases. Faith has a big part in curing cancer.

At that time the word "cancer" was a very bad word. I saw many people who just gave up when they found out they had cancer. It seemed to me, and it has been borne out in research, that this hastened their going downhill and dying. Some people who were expected to do well, based on the medical facts, did poorly, and some who were expected to do poorly, did well. We all saw cases that defied medical expectations. A patient predicted not to live more than a few days might live on in order to see a daughter married or a child born or somebody graduate from college. They lived far longer than we thought they possibly could. I was impressed by how much power the mind seemed to have in these settings.

One of the things we frequently faced was relatives telling us, "Don't tell Mom that she's got cancer. She won't be able to stand it."

I am seeing now that when one didn't discuss the cancer, it really hurt the patient's chances of recovery and frequently hurt the family. If she was not going to recover, it hurt her last days, because everybody was living a sham and pretending that there was nothing the matter.

In one or two cases, when I finished an operation and went off to tell the family that we had found cancer, the family would say, "Oh now, you mustn't tell Mother. You mustn't tell Mother. She couldn't stand it. Don't say anything to her about it."

Then the next morning when I would go in to see the patient, she would call me over next to the bed and say, "Now I know you found cancer, and I know it is bad, but you mustn't tell my family because they wouldn't be able to stand it."

This cultural attitude made the last days very difficult for everybody. Nowadays we try to get the patient and family to discuss it openly. In the first place, the family needs to be convinced that many people are cured of cancer—more and more every day. It is important to stress that it is not something to just give up and get out the blue suit and get it pressed. Patients, and families as well, have a much better life if it is an open situation.

Today, clinicians are required to tell the patient everything and that is a good thing. One could hardly give someone chemotherapy without telling them what it is for. It is such a drastic treatment. Now there are laws about informed consent. The patient has to be told exactly what is planned and what complications or side effects there may be. Sometimes this is not all good because in telling patients about anything that is possible, even though most of them are extremely improbable, the patients might get so scared that they wonder if they ought to have the treatment.

During the worst of the oral contraception litigation in California, a state which led the country for years in malpractice cases, the insurance companies wanted doctors to tell everybody to whom they gave birth control pills what the complications might be. It turned out there were 80 or more possible complications of the birth control pill, almost all of which were never seen. Nobody had enough time to sit down and go over 80 complications every time they wrote a prescription for birth control pills.

The business of telling people what they have and in some way telling them what to expect is far better now than what used to go on. Conveying unpleasant news can be done in different ways, sometimes in a very bad way and sometimes in a good one. For instance, a physician might find a very advanced cancer and say to that patient, "Well, this is really bad, and it looks as if you're probably not going to survive for more than a month or two." An alternative is to say to the patient, "Things are very grave, but everything will be done to see if the condition can be improved. There is so much research going on. We don't know what might come along. In six months to a year what is hopeless today might be able to be completely cured. I try not to take hope away even in the worst situations. When I started practice, no one ever lived a year with a placental malignancy called choriocarcinoma no matter what we did. It was the first cancer to respond dramatically to chemotherapy. In six months time, the prognosis changed from a 100% mortality to a 98% cure rate. Hodgkins disease is another that used to be 100% fatal. Now it is almost 100% cured. After I moved to Asheville, I saw a 14-year-old girl with Hodgkins disease who later married and had children.

I believe that telling people how long they are going to live is a very bad mistake. Most of us with experience have found that out. Many, many patients, who have been told they have a month to live, have lived for some years. I had a patient to whom I didn't give such a prediction, despite her poor prognosis. I operated on her in the early 1950s and found a very far advanced cancer of the ovary. With a long, complicated operation, I was able to get out all that I could see, but in far-advanced cancer of the ovary, frequently the peritoneal fluid has cells in it. These microscopic cells will float around in there and eventually attach to something, and the patient will come down with a recurrence. She had a spot of cancer on the bowel and along the side of the pelvis. I told her husband after the operation that the cancer had been very far advanced and I doubted very much if I got it all, and I wouldn't be surprised if she didn't have a recurrence within six months. That was in 1953, and she is alive and well with no evidence of cancer today. So I learned that lesson early.

It is the other extreme not to tell the patient anything. I don't remember ever doing this, but with some patients, surgeons would open up the abdomen and not be able to do very much, and close the abdomen. The patient wouldn't know (all she had was a scar) if she wasn't told anything. She wouldn't know what had transpired, what the diagnosis was or the possible outcome. She would not have the opportunity to take control of her remaining days and put her affairs in order.

At the time I left the Norburn Clinic and started in practice for myself, obstetrics was entirely different from the way it is now. Hospitals in the city of Asheville were delivering about 3500 patients a year, and most were delivered by general practitioners. There were eight doctors in town, including myself, who called themselves specialists and limited their practices to obstetrics and gynecology. Four of us were either board-certified or board-eligible as specialists, having passed our examinations or having been about ready to take them, and three were doctors who had some extra training in obstetrics and gynecology but called themselves specialists. In addition, there was one general practitioner who treated his patients very well, was highly respected and delivered several hundred babies a year while continuing to do general practice. He knew when to refer to an Ob/Gyn specialist. When some of the general practitioners in the community had a patient who needed a cesarean section, they would call general surgeons rather than the trained obstetricians.

Through the years, the number of general practitioners—and later, family practitioners—doing obstetrics decreased steadily. It wasn't a good financial situation for the family practitioners because they didn't charge high fees and they couldn't afford to be out of their office five or six hours attending to someone in labor. Their office was their main source of income. They wanted to do obstetrics because they wanted to have the family stay with them. When they delivered the baby, they would expect to take care of it, and the child would become another one of their regular patients. They felt they might lose the whole family if they didn't do the delivery and then the baby was seen by a pediatrician. At the present time, there are very few family practitioners in the Asheville area delivering babies.

Fees in those days were extremely modest compared to now. Most obstetricians charged about $150 for prenatal care and delivery and one postpartum visit. A lot of us, including me, were happy if we only received $100 in some circumstances.

I remember that one enterprising young man just starting his family came to me to discuss his wife's costs. When I quoted him $150, he said that he would pay cash right then if I would take 10% off, which I was glad to do. Fees rose rather slowly over the first few years of practice. We started at $100 to $150. In the mid 60s we were still getting $200 to $250.

In our group we were at $250 for delivery and prenatal care when one of the other doctors—new in town—started in at $300. Some of the people around me wanted to go to $300 also, but I thought it was better to stay at $250 for the patient's sake. In those days, insurance paid very little for obstetrics. Most insurance companies—and even the insurance for industry—paid only $30 to $50 for delivery. The burden of the fees fell upon the individuals. Most of our practice was made up of women married to middle class workers—such as plumbers and painters—so I stayed at $250. Then Nixon put in a price freeze so that nobody could raise fees. This lasted for 18 months. So there I was, stuck at $250 when some of the other men, even the ones who were not trained nearly as well as I, were getting considerably more.

Quite a few of the doctors charged extra if they had to do a cesarean section. I never did that because I didn't want there to be any question about whether I might have done a cesarean that wasn't absolutely necessary in order to get a higher fee.

Today, vaginal delivery and cesarean births cost several thousand dollars. One of the reasons for higher fees in obstetrics is the way malpractice premiums have escalated.

Malpractice claims in those days were considerably less frequent than now. People were not looking to sue. There were very, very few lawsuits. It is almost unbelievable in this day and age that the first malpractice premium that I paid was $29 for a year. I had only $5,000 worth of insurance because nobody ever sued anybody for the amounts that are routine today. When I stopped practice in 1985, Asheville doctors who were doing obstetrics were paying $40,000 per year in malpractice premiums. At the time of publication of this book, this has risen to over $200,000 in some locations in the country.

Besides the deliveries of our private practice, we also had to deliver welfare clinic patients. These were patients who came to the hospital with no doctor and no money. We took call in rotation for their care. For a long time, there were 14 of us doing this. We took one 24-hour-call duty every 14 days. I remember at one point I was delivering a clinic patient when one of my private patients delivered in bed in the labor room. Fortunately, she was not unhappy about that.

The office practice of obstetrics was much simpler in the early days. For instance, laboratory tests were quite few. We did a routine complete blood count and urine on the patient and an Rh test at the first prenatal visit. The Rh factor test had just come into being a very few years earlier and was not as complicated at that time. The pregnancy test was not as common as it is now. The only pregnancy test we had was the so-called rabbit test, which was complex and expensive. The test consisted of taking the patient's urine and injecting it into the vein of a rabbit. Two days later the rabbit was sacrificed, and if the ovary showed ovulation, then the patient was pregnant because the hormones in her urine were such that it would stimulate the rabbit to ovulate. Of course, this was not done in the office. Laboratories kept the rabbits. Because it was not a very efficient test at all, with the need to sacrifice a rabbit for every test, few were done. It was only if a complication was suspected—like an ectopic pregnancy or to seek a reason why a woman was not menstruating—and the clinical examination was equivocal about whether she was pregnant or not, that a physician ordered the test.

Now, the laboratory pregnancy tests are extremely simple, almost like a litmus test, and there is largely a reliance on ultrasound to tell whether there is a pregnancy in the uterus or not.

We seldom did X-rays unless, toward the end of pregnancy, we suspected twins and wanted to be sure or if we suspected a fetal abnormality. Sometimes in extremely obese people, when it was impossible to be sure of feeling anything, we took an X-ray to see if the patient was pregnant. She had to be at least four months along for the fetus to show up on the X-ray. We also used X-ray to see if the pelvic inlet was large enough for the baby to go through in the birth process. We could measure the pelvic size indirectly with our examining fingers in a pelvic examination, typically done at the patient's first visit, but the X-ray, usually done at term if there was a concern, was much more accurate. We were appropriately concerned that too much X-raying of the abdomen during pregnancy might lead to problems of the fetus. There is some evidence that too many X-rays might bring on a form of leukemia after the baby is born or might even cause a malformation.

In infertility work, one of the tests available was designed to see if the fallopian tubes were open so that the eggs and sperm could get together. Ordinarily we did that with air, specifically carbon dioxide. We put air with pressure up through the uterus with a cannula in the cervix and determined the pressure required for the air to go through the tube into the abdominal cavity. If the tube seemed to be blocked, using a form of continuous X-ray called fluoroscopy, dye was injected into the uterus and we watched it go through the tube to see where it was blocked. This allowed us to decide whether or not the problem could be repaired surgically.

I had as patients two sisters, both of whom were infertile. I couldn't get air through the tubes of one of them, so I did a dye test on her. We always did this in the first two weeks of the menstrual cycle so that we were sure that the patient couldn't be pregnant at the time. Apparently the dye unblocked her tubes because she got pregnant right after the test. Her sister, whose tubes were open to the air test, kept insisting that we do the dye test on her, too. I kept telling her that we didn't need to do one because her tubes were open. After her sister got pregnant, she was just adamant that she have the test. I thought, well it won't do her any harm. I consented to do the test late in the cycle because it was the only time she could have it. She never had another period. She was obviously pregnant at the time of the test because we did it after her fertile period, the ovulation period. The rest of her nine months I held my breath hoping that the fluoroscopy had not damaged the baby. Fortunately, she had a very healthy baby and I was relieved. She didn't know that I was worrying for the whole nine months.

A woman in her 40s, who had had her family in her 20s, developed a lot of trouble with her stomach. She was not my patient at the time. She was having nausea and indigestion and went to one of the very good internists in town who proceeded to do a variety of gastric X-rays to see what was wrong with her stomach. Finally she ended up in my office where I diagnosed a three-month pregnancy. That was the reason for her nausea. We held our breaths for the rest of her pregnancy, wondering if the fluoroscopy had damaged her baby. Again, it had not. The baby appeared perfectly normal, much to my relief.

Today, with the use of ultrasound, it is rare to perform an X-ray for concerns related to pregnancy. In addition, there are now many other blood tests done routinely in pregnancy.

There are several congenital diseases, which we knew little about in the 1940s and 1950s, but although relatively uncommon, some of them could have been treated if they had been detected extremely early. Now mothers are screened for some genetic conditions during mid-pregnancy. We have learned that lack of folic acid is associated with some congenital defects such as spinal bifida, and therefore, we make sure that the mothers have an adequate intake of folic acid in their diet and in vitamins. If they are of reproductive age, we advise them to take it ahead of the time that conception might occur.

By the mid 1950s, my practice had grown to be large and time-consuming. I had a solo practice at that time, sharing an office with another obstetrician. We helped each other by assisting on operations, and when one person was out of town, the other one took his calls. But we did not step in for each other on a regular basis. Most of the time, we took care of our own patients—regardless of when they called us.

In those days, we worked a long week. I tried to take Thursday afternoons off. On Saturdays, the office was open in the morning, and the patients liked this very much, because sometimes the husband wanted to come with the patient, and he wouldn't have to get off work. Other offices began to close Saturday mornings and do a five-day week long before we did. In fact, I think our office was the last one in town to have Saturday morning office hours.

I felt that the advantages of practicing solo were very great. I got to know my patients, and they got to know me. We got along very well together. This helped in taking care of them because I knew what their family situations were and their emotional problems—if any. Sometimes, I could anticipate problems because I knew how the patient was going to react to situations in her life. The disadvantage of solo practice was that it was very hard on my family. As I got busier in obstetrics, I was up many nights. Sometimes five and six nights would go by in a row when I wouldn't sleep the whole night through. I can remember many occasions when I would go to bed at 7:30 p.m. so if I got called at 12 or 12:30 a.m., I would have had a pretty fair night's sleep.

The old adage that most babies are born at night is not particularly true, but almost every patient who went into labor disturbed my sleep, either because she called and went into the hospital at night and delivered in the daytime, or she called in the day and delivered at night. Either way, I had to get up and go check and see how she was doing. I enjoyed practicing, and if a physician enjoys what he or she is doing, it is possible to work very hard without generating any serious health problems.

Practice of Obstetrics

Obstetrics was a good specialty for me because it dealt with younger people who by and large were quite happy. People were glad and pleased with the result when things went well—and things usually went well. There were times when a pregnancy was not a happy situation. If we had a baby with a serious congenital problem, that was a disaster for the parents, of course, but there were also other types of sadness. I remember to this day a 22-year-old from a wealthy family in a city about 1500 – 2000 miles from Asheville. I was called by her doctor in that city who said that she was pregnant and single and that her folks wanted her to come to Asheville and stay during the pregnancy so that their friends would not know anything about it. The plan would be for her to deliver in Asheville and have the baby adopted. I accepted taking care of her. She came with her mother when she was about five months pregnant and stayed in a hotel the whole time.

During the time of the prenatal visits, I got to know her well. She was a very attractive person, a college graduate, and she seemed to me to be extremely intelligent. She had become engaged to a man and, at some point during the engagement, had missed a period. Before she could tell him she thought she was pregnant, he came to her and broke the engagement, saying he had fallen in love with someone else. She never told him she was pregnant with his child but went on and had the baby, and we had it adopted into a family in another city. They were also very intelligent people, and we knew they would bring the child up well.

Two or three days after she delivered, before she left the hospital, I went to her room, and she was crying. I asked if I could help. She unburdened herself that she had loved this man so much and had lost him, and now she had his baby whom she had to give up. It was a very touching situation, and I always wondered what happened both to the baby and to her. I hoped that she met someone else and eventually had more children and had a good life. I give the girl great credit for not trying to force the man to marry her, even though I know there are people who might disagree with me.

Another case was entirely different from this one in that, instead of craving the baby she had lost, my patient rejected the baby she kept. I performed the delivery of a clinic patient—a charity patient on the welfare service. She already had six boys, and when she was told she had a seventh boy, she began to rant and rave that she didn't want anything to do with him; she wouldn't see him. She said her six boys were nothing but trouble, and she couldn't stand another one. She literally refused to take the baby home. We had quite a time getting her to accept the seventh boy and finally persuaded her to take him home. I've wondered how that poor little fella grew up in that family.

Sometimes the same situation will get two different responses. I had one patient who had four children. Her husband was a businessman whose work was not giving him a very good living. She became pregnant for the fifth time and was perfectly willing to have the baby and really thought it was okay. I missed the fact that she had twins. Missing twins was not unusual in those days. Much to my surprise, when she came to deliver, I delivered two perfectly healthy babies. I knew I had to tell the father that he had twins. I thought this would make him unhappy, since I knew he was having financial problems, and this would add to his burden. I went out to the waiting room, took a deep breath and told him, expecting him to be upset that I hadn't known that she was going to have twins. He was extremely happy. He thought that was just the greatest thing in the world—to have two babies instead of one.

Another patient had four or five children and a husband who didn't keep a job at all. I suspect he drank quite a bit. She had to work very hard to support the babies. About five or six months into the pregnancy, I suspected that she had twins. She was working at one of the hospitals, and I sent her down to get an X-ray to see whether she indeed had two fetuses. I went to the radiology department with her, and several people who worked with her were also present. Everybody was filled with anticipation. When we held the X-ray up and showed that she did have two babies, the friends were all ecstatic, jumping up and down and congratulating her. She stood over on one side with her head down and tears running down her face. I knew that she was overwhelmed by the fact that she was going to have to work all the harder to keep the family together and supply for two more babies instead of one more.

I was consulted by an Asheville factory worker in her early twenties. She came in with a complaint that her periods had stopped. She was single. I took a history and examined her. It was obvious that she was five or six months pregnant. She seemed not to have the slightest idea what was the matter with her. After the examination, we went back into the office and I explained to her that she was pregnant and predicted the time she might expect to deliver. I then told her that she had several options. She could have the baby and keep it or have the baby and then have it adopted. I could send her down to Charlotte where there was a Florence Crittenton Home. If she so chose, she could go to Charlotte right then and live there until the baby was delivered. They would have the baby adopted, and she could come home without too many people knowing about it. After explaining all of this to her, I said, "What about marrying the fellow?"

She said, "I would not marry him; he is the most awful person!" And she went on to say over and over how terrible he was, and the horrible things he did.

I could not stand it any longer so I said, "Well if he is that bad, why did you have intercourse with him?"

She said, "Oh, he kept insisting . . . you know how men are."

A patient in her mid thirties came to me for obstetrical care. Her husband had always been working, so I had never met him. After the delivery, I went to the waiting room, and there was an older man with white hair, whom I estimated to be about 60 years of age. "Are you with Mrs. Jones?" I asked.

"Yes," he replied.

"You have a nice grandson."

He drew himself up. "That's my baby."

I never made that mistake again.

A fairly young married woman came in with a new pregnancy. Early in the prenatal course, she was diagnosed with a very severe cancer. The time came to review her treatment options. She was told that she could be given chemotherapy, which would be lethal to the baby, and she would probably miscarry. This would prolong her life some but would not cure her. Her alternative was to have the baby, forgoing immediate treatment. This choice would probably shorten her life. She entered into the discussion. After considerable thinking on her part, and I suppose talking at length with her husband, she decided that if she was going to die anyway, a few extra months were not enough to compensate for the loss of her baby, and she would like to leave her baby alive and well. So she went through the pregnancy with no treatment for her disease and delivered a healthy, full-term baby girl. She had two weeks with her newborn, holding and feeding her. Then she died. I always thought she was a very courageous person and certainly had to go through a lot in making her choice. It affected all of us who had anything to do with her, because she kept her spirits up after the baby was born. She was very happy with the short time with her baby. It set an example for everybody.

I delivered quite a few ministers' wives, and in doing so, I came to realize what a difficult life most of them had. They would tell me their problems. Many of them lived in a fishbowl, or thought they did. One minister with a church out in the country lived in a house right next door. The church did not have a kitchen in it, so it was not uncommon for ladies to come into the home unannounced to take over the kitchen to prepare a luncheon for some group. This bothered the minister's wife considerably, as I imagine most women can understand.

Another wife of a minister came from a fairly wealthy family in another city. She was used to having all the amenities and suddenly found herself in a small house out in the country near her husband's small church where he had started his pastorate. They were enjoying their healthy baby, but she had considerable trouble adjusting to the life they had to lead. When they were transferred after a while to another church some distance away, I hoped they got along better.

I had as a patient the wife of a minister of a fairly large church in the Asheville area. She had delivered three children and had to work very hard at raising them, along with her other obligations. The couple couldn't afford help, and the husband was absorbed in his church work and didn't seem to realize what a job she had. With her fourth baby, she went into labor about 11 o'clock on Saturday night. I met them at the hospital. The minister complained rather bitterly to me that she had gone into labor on Saturday night. He had to preach in the morning, and he didn't appreciate the fact that he couldn't get any rest. She delivered about 3 o'clock Sunday morning, and when we took her into her room, he was in her bed sound asleep. We had to get him out of the bed before we could put her in it. I had to keep after him after that to stop trying to make her do so much church work.

The parishioners expected her to be teaching Sunday School, making shut-in calls, and at the same time, taking care of her rapidly growing family. All of this was overwhelming. It gave me an understanding that ministers' wives sometimes have to be the angels in the family and put up with a great deal in order for the husbands to be successful ministers.

RURAL MEDICINE

As I look back on my obstetrical practice, I think of some individual cases that were referred to me by family practitioners out in the country and in the mountains. Some of the cases were extremely interesting and challenging. It is a great pleasure to reflect on the events and see that I have helped some people who were in bad shape when they were referred.

One of the doctors out in the mountains sent in a patient having her first baby prematurely. She was 32 or 33, which in those days was quite late in life for a pregnant woman. Nowadays, it is a common age for a woman to have her first baby. She was about six months pregnant when she had gone into labor. She had planned to have a home delivery, but she just didn't deliver. The doctor couldn't determine why and finally sent her in.

On examination, I found that she had a large cervical fibroid, a non-malignant tumor the size of a baseball, originating in the upper cervix ahead of the baby, and the baby couldn't get past it. So I started to do a cesarean on her and take out the fibroid. When I opened the abdomen, I saw she had seven large fibroids in the muscles all through the uterus. Ordinarily, I would have taken the uterus out but it was her only pregnancy, and it was obvious this baby was not going to live. It was too premature. I wanted to preserve her ability to have children if I could, so I did seven myomyectomies on her, meaning that there were seven scars in her uterus in areas where the fibroids had been evacuated. One fibroid went far into the uterine cavity so I went on into that area and took the fibroid out and extracted the baby through that incision. The baby died right away. The mother recovered very well. While she was in the hospital, I kept counseling her that if she got pregnant again, she must get good obstetrical care immediately because she had those seven incisions in her uterus and one of them could rupture as the uterus got bigger.

The next time I saw her was two years later when I was on call for charity patients at St. Josephs. I had received a call that there was a patient who had been sent in by a midwife from Madison County because she had been in labor for three days. I went in to see her. I remember that it was in the middle of the night. I took one look at her and realized this was the woman whom I had counseled to be so careful of the scars in the uterus for fear they would rupture. Here she had been in labor for three solid days! I immediately took her to the operating room and did a cesarean on her and got her a live baby. It was amazing that all those scars held up as well as they did. I must say that although she didn't take my advice, she got along surprisingly well without it.

One day a man called me on a Sunday with a very aggrieved voice. I could tell he was really hurt. "Doc, you sent me a dun!"

The first time I was told this, I did not know what it meant. I began to ask around to the doctors in the county, and, over time, they and the country folk explained it to me. I had to learn not to send bills to certain of my patients. They were doing the best they could. I had come from the cities, and, in keeping with the systems I had learned, sent a bill every month to everyone who owed the practice money.

The people in some of the rural counties around us didn't have money. There was a whole system for seeing doctors. A lot of my patients came down from there. They typically had three or four acres they lived on—with a cow, a pig and chickens—and they raised corn. These were for their sustenance. In addition, they often had about an acre and a half of tobacco. That crop provided the only cash they had for the whole year.

They sold the tobacco crop in November. When they got their $1500 cash for tobacco, they'd come around to the office, even though the surgery may have been ten months earlier, and would peel out what they saw as our portion of the cash—perhaps 30 or 50 dollars.

The physician was not expected to send any additional bills. That was it. They used that method every time they owed money. The arrangement lasted until the next year. As I learned the system, I gradually knew whom in my practice I should bill and whom not to bill.

I didn't have anything to do with the male midwives out in one of the rural counties because they never sent me any patients, but one of the very fine and very busy family practitioners used to get most of their calls for help when they found themselves in the middle of a problem they couldn't handle. He would send the patients on to me. Apparently, there were three male midwives without specific training . . . correction . . . without any formal training. Yet they did go around and deliver babies.

A colleague told me a story—the validity of which is left to doubt—that reveals some of the disdain for unqualified caregivers. A male midwife who was going away for vacation, had a patient about to deliver. He couldn't find anybody to cover for him so he enlisted a man who was not a trained veterinarian but who did a lot of work with animals. The man liked animals and took care of them while they were sick. The midwife convinced him to be his stand-by to deliver the baby. As it happened, the midwife was away when the baby came, and when the midwife got back and asked the "veterinarian" how things had gone, the man said, "I'm never gonna do this again; it's a terrible thing. The baby was born okay, but I had a terrible time after that. It took me two hours to get her to eat the placenta, and I had to lick the baby dry myself."

PREECLAMPSIA/ECLAMPSIA

We used to get quite a few eclamptic patients—three or four a year. These were women, such as I saw in my residency, with preeclampsia so severe that they would go into convulsions. The typical symptoms are that the patient's blood pressure starts to rise and albumen appears in the urine. Usually, it is a fairly slow process and can be treated as preeclampsia before eclampsia develops. At that time, eclampsia was a very dangerous thing, and some of the women died from it. It usually did not occur in people who had good prenatal care but was not uncommon in women who did not seek prenatal care. It wasn't that the family practitioners didn't supply it, but that the people didn't come in . . . until they were getting desperately ill with preeclampsia in the last three months of pregnancy. There were some new treatments coming along for these patients, such as intravenous magnesium sulfate, which helped a great deal. By and large, if treatment was instigated in a timely way, the outcomes for these women were very successful.

In a case of eclampsia, besides the patient having convulsions, her liver could be badly affected. There could be hemorrhaging into the tissues such that the liver would actually shut down. Most times, areas of the placenta died. Frequently, the baby would die of a lack of oxygen and nutrients because of the loss of placental function. The condition is limited to the pregnancy, so the treatment for severe cases is still to this day to terminate the pregnancy either by vaginal delivery or cesarean section. Then, ordinarily, the patient will gradually recover without having aftereffects. Occasionally, liver or kidney damage persists after the pregnancy, but this is rare. I remember one patient that died because of the eclampsia and another patient who died because the high blood pressure was so severe that she ruptured an aneurysm in her brain.

There was a great deal of study of toxemia from the 1930s on through the 1960s and some interesting things came out. One of them was that it seemed to be more frequent in certain months of the year. March was a month in which it was very prevalent. There was another study that showed that when there was a great deal of toxemia in one part of the world, that was also the case in other parts of the world. When Europe was seeing quite a lot of toxemia, so was India. It seemed to go in waves or clusters, and nobody knew exactly why.

PLACENTAL ABRUPTION

One of the most interesting cases I remember involved what is called placental abruption. This is a situation in which the placenta suddenly separates from the uterine wall. Sometimes it occurred with labor, but, more commonly, this could occur without labor. The risk of the condition is increased with toxemia. The separation could be partial where a part of the placenta remains connected, or it could involve the whole placenta. Bleeding occurs because the blood vessels from the mother going into the placenta are torn. The resulting hemorrhage can be extremely heavy. In this particular instance, I was called by a Canton family practitioner—a very good one. He needed me to come right out to the hospital where he had a patient four-and-one-half months pregnant and bleeding heavily. By the time I got there, I was able to extract the baby as a breech and get the placenta out. The bleeding stopped, and the patient recovered well.

The next time I saw the patient, she was bleeding at about seven months with a new pregnancy. Her doctor put her into an ambulance and sent her to Asheville. She had a premature separation and was able to deliver vaginally. The baby died because it was too premature. A year or two later, he again sent the same patient over with a more advanced separation, and the whole process happened quicker. The baby was dead by the time she arrived at the hospital. She lost so much blood before and after delivery, she eventually required eleven transfusions in order to bring her blood count up to normal.

When she got pregnant again, he asked me if I would take her over and do her prenatal care. The patient was a very intelligent woman, and by this time, she knew quite a bit about the disease of premature separation. None of us had ever seen it occur serially as she had been experiencing.

We took diligent care of her during the fourth pregnancy and saw her very frequently. A researcher at Bowman Gray Medical School heard about her and was interested in her case. During the last six weeks of pregnancy, we collected special urine specimens and sent them to the university research laboratory. The investigator checked the levels of serotonin, which is a product made in nerve cells and excreted in the urine. He was interested in seeing whether a drop in serotonin could cause premature separation of the placenta.

She was very cooperative. Once a week, she would save all her urine for 24 hours, and we would send it down there for him to check. I had warned her of the very early symptoms of a placental abruption. When she was about eight months pregnant, she called and said she had a severe backache, one of the warning signs. I told her to get to the hospital as fast as she could. While she was en route, I rallied a team for a cesarean section set up. They were ready to go when she got to the emergency room and we did a very rapid operative delivery. At that time, she was not bleeding; she still had only a severe backache. Some of my colleagues thought I was a little bit nuts to be doing an emergency cesarean for a backache. By the time we got into the abdomen, we could see the blood streaks flaring out through the uterine muscle. I was extremely happy for this woman to get a live baby because she had gone through so much trying to have one.

I wrote this case up and presented it to the North Carolina Obstetrical and Gynecological Society where it created quite a stir and comments from the professors at Duke and Bowman Gray. When we finally got the serotonin report back from the urine sample that was taken the day before she separated her placenta, the serotonin level had dropped. This fact was of great interest to people doing research in that area of medicine.

ABDOMINAL PREGNANCY

It is an exceedingly rare event for a woman to develop a fetus outside the pelvic organs. However, over the years of my practice, I encountered four women with this life-threatening condition in which the fertilized egg, instead of going up into the tube and into the uterus, drops into the abdominal cavity and grows there. This probably happens much more frequently than we know. Usually, the fertilized egg doesn't implant and dies because it has no blood supply or oxygen. But occasionally, when it gets into the abdominal cavity, it will fall into a place where there is some blood supply near the surface, and it will implant there and grow. The placenta grows around the intestines and other abdominal organs and is thus able to feed the baby. Frequently, abdominal pregnancies don't reach full term because the placenta is inadequate for that.

Making the diagnosis can be challenging. If the pregnancy is full-term, it is not too difficult. On examination of the patient, there is no uterus between the clinician's hands and the fetus. The baby is essentially right under the skin. It feels different. Before ultrasonography came into common clinical usage, an X-ray of the abdomen would show that there were loops of intestines around the baby, unlike when the baby is in the uterus. Abdominal pregnancies require operation. It is usually critically important to operate whenever the diagnosis is made because of the grave danger of trying to let the patient carry to term.

One of my patients with an abdominal pregnancy was at four months when we discovered it. It was necessary to operate immediately and take out the fetus. The cardinal law of operating on women with this condition is not to take out the placenta. If the placenta is peeled off the abdominal organs, wherever it is implanted, it leaves open very large blood vessels from the body. It is almost impossible to stop the bleeding and the patient can very well bleed to death. The body is an amazing instrument. If the umbilical cord is tied off very close to the placenta—very gingerly so as not to dislodge any of it—in some months, the placenta will be absorbed, and, if the patient is operated on again for another reason, there won't be any evidence of the placenta.

Two of the patients sent to me were full-term, and we successfully diagnosed the abdominal pregnancies, operated on them and got living babies. The third case didn't turn out as well. I was called to see a woman when her physician thought she was in labor because she had a lot of abdominal pain. He wanted to know if I thought she would deliver vaginally. I did a pelvic examination on her and found the cervix to be closed. I didn't pick up the fact that there was any difference in her abdominal examination. I thought that she was just having some false labor with this pain. I was called to see her again a couple of days later, and I made the diagnosis of abdominal pregnancy and did an immediate cesarean. The baby was dead and had been for some time, but the placenta was over in the right side of the abdomen and had moved down. While I was tying the cord off so that we could remove the baby and leave the placenta, suddenly one of the vessels connecting the placenta to the woman's body ruptured, and we were faced with a massive hemorrhage. There was no way of getting down and trying to ligate that vessel because it was under the placenta, and I felt that if I did that, I would simply knock more of the placenta off, and the patient would surely bleed to death.

I put a pack on the vessel with pressure and held it for about twenty minutes, hoping that a clot would form and we could remove the pack and leave the placenta where it was, but when I removed the pack, she started to bleed again very heavily.

I repacked it and, after seeing that the vessel was not going to close off by itself, I sewed the pack in place in order to control the bleeding, hoping that after two or three days we could take out the pack and she would not hemorrhage again. She did stabilize over three days, and I re-operated on her. I took the pack out and she bled a little, but not very much, and we sewed her up. We had her on antibiotics at that time but she began spiking a fever. Culture showed that she had an anaerobic infection—one in which the bacteria thrive in the absence of oxygen. At that time, we didn't have any good antibiotics for such virulent organisms, although we gave her one that sometimes worked. For a time, it helped, but then her condition worsened, and after about thirty days, she succumbed to the infection.

BREECH

One of the changes that has happened in obstetrics is the general philosophy concerning the manner of delivery of a breech. Concern about safety of vaginal delivery has been resolved in most places by delivering almost all breeches by cesarean section. Why not do a cesarean on all of them? The main problem is that it is more of an operation. In general, cesarean sections have a greater complication rate than vaginal deliveries despite modern hospital facilities with well-supplied blood banks. The woman can occasionally get a pulmonary embolism, contract an infection that is difficult to cure—even with modern antibiotics—or suffer effects of anesthesia mishaps. Another significant problem is that with a cesarean, a scar is left on the uterus, which has the potential of rupturing in future pregnancies. This could become an extremely serious situation.

I remember going to one meeting of the North Carolina Obstetrical and Gynecological Society of which I was president. There was a report on delivering breeches by cesareans, stating that it was the only way to manage a breech. At the same meeting, there was a report from the North Carolina Maternal Mortality Committee, which by state law checks all maternal deaths in North Carolina each year and files reports on them. There had been four maternal mortalities the year before from ruptured cesarean section scars. If a breech can be delivered normally through the pelvis, there is some reason to consider it; however, nowadays there are almost none delivered vaginally.

There is another disadvantage to this liberal use of surgery for breech delivery. Future obstetricians do not acquire skills in vaginal delivery of breeches. If a woman comes in the hospital in labor with a breech ready to deliver, even the highest trained obstetricians would, in the future, essentially have no experience at delivering her fetus vaginally as a breech. Several times in the latter part of my practice, I would be in the labor room when a woman came in ready to deliver a breech, and her obstetrician was a younger man who had been trained to section all patients in this setting. But there was obviously no time to prepare for the cesarean. He would call me in to help him with the technical challenges of the delivery because he didn't feel competent to do it.

Just as in my residency, during the first few years of my obstetrical practice, I tried to deliver most breeches through the pelvis as a normal delivery. Because I had performed many breech deliveries in my training, I had become quite proficient at it. Back then, we performed very few cesareans, and so it was always a matter of great deliberation if we considered a cesarean section for a breech. I never failed to remember my residency teaching that attempting vaginal delivery of a breech could get a physician into serious trouble. Entrapment of the head—occurring when the smaller-diameter body slips through a pelvis too small for the head to follow—could result in hemorrhages in the child's brain if any degree of force must be applied to get the head through. Prolapse of the umbilical cord—if the membranes ruptured during labor and the breech was not down against the pelvic inlet—would require working very rapidly to get the baby out before the cord was compressed and the baby's oxygen supply was cut off. A nuchal arm—an arm trapped behind the head—would require maneuvers skillfully performed to get the arm down in the correct position so that it didn't cause trouble.

There were many criteria we used to decide whether or not to deliver a breech from below. One, of course, was the size of the pelvis. Both from an internal examination and from X-ray pelvimetry, we could determine fairly accurately the dimensions of the bony passage that the baby would need to transverse. If it was smaller than normal, we didn't take any chances.

Another factor that caused us to watch closely was whether or not labor had progressed well. Just as I had learned at Harvard, it was a fairly good rule that if labor progressed rapidly and normally, the baby was a size that could be delivered from below. Typically, a fetus would not push a good fast labor unless it was deliverable.

PAIN CONTROL

One of the major changes in the practice of obstetrics through the years was the change in pain control during labor and during delivery. When I started practice, the idea was to "knock out the woman" in labor so that she did not remember any pain. This state was commonly called twilight sleep and was induced by various combinations of drugs. As was true of the majority of practices in those years, in my observation, the women in my practice all expected to have good medication for pain and didn't know much about the labor—and didn't want to. They thought it was great to wake up and discover the baby was there, no problems, as long as it was safe. The technique had been proven to be safe.

We did do some spinal anesthesia for the actual deliveries. That was administered by people who knew what they were doing. Most obstetricians, in fact, had been trained to do spinals. We simply gave a very low dose of a type of drug like Novocain into the spinal column. It was heavier than the spinal fluid so it sank to the bottom of the column when the patient was sitting up. A few minutes after it was administered, it was bound to the nerves at that lower area, and it was then safe for her to lie down. That produced a very small but adequate area of anesthesia, just the pelvic area. It was quite effective and had essentially no risk of harm to the baby. It did have the disadvantage that some people got rather severe headaches after it.

Then for a short time, there was popularized a pain-relief method called presacral anesthesia. The anesthetic was injected into some holes in the sacral bone. The medication went upward into the spinal column and affected the nerves going to the pelvis. This, in competent hands, was also effective, although it was a little challenging to administer. People started performing the procedure who were not trained in it, and there were several deaths from putting the needle in too far and piercing the dura which surrounds the spinal cord. The anesthesia would, in that case, go up the spinal cord and affect the woman's breathing.

Then, about 1960, the advocacy of so-called natural childbirth started. Women attended classes and were told how to relax. The husband was there and learned about it also. Together they practiced going through labor and practiced breathing techniques to be performed during the pains. The woman had to do without any anesthesia at all. This got to be quite a popular thing, and a great many people wanted it. We had classes, usually started by a woman who was personally very interested in it, and some of the doctors sent their patients.

One of the difficulties I found with this was that the people running the courses were extreme advocates of it, and they pushed it very hard. Some of the patients felt that if they didn't go through the whole birth without anything for pain, they had failed. We observed this over and over and found it rather tragic.

The reason for going to an obstetrician in the first place is not for a normal delivery, it is to take care of any problems that might arise. Sometimes, problems arise very rapidly in labor, and the physician has to move quickly to get a successful outcome. Sometimes, a woman just cannot deliver vaginally for one reason or another and has to have a cesarean. I had one patient who had attended these classes on natural childbirth whose labor progressed very slowly. Finally, after a full 24 hours in labor, it became obvious that she could not deliver vaginally and that the baby was getting into jeopardy. I explained the situation and the need for a cesarean delivery to her husband and to her. The couple acquiesced without any problem, but after the delivery, during the rest of the time that she was in the hospital, she was extremely depressed. It was her first baby and everything had gone well. The baby was fine and she was fine, but she kept saying to me every time I came in, "Where did I fail? I'm a failure; I didn't have this baby the way I should have."

It was difficult seeing people get into this problem. I always felt it was a failure of the natural birth classes not to tell the people that they might have to have an intervention of one kind or the other and that it wasn't their fault. Most doctors I knew would tell their patients, "Go ahead and start it, but if you get so you want something for the pain, we will give it to you. You don't have to go through this." This infuriated certain of the women who were running the classes. So at times, it was almost a battle between some of the physicians and some of the educators. There were also disagreements concerning what pregnancy was, how the baby developed and the husband's role. I never was keen on the idea that the husband should be right there during the delivery. Frankly, I didn't understand why a husband wanted to see a delivery. But, if he did, it was all right with me if the wife wanted him there.

I got into a little trouble over this with the husband of one of my patients. I had done quite a bit of wild animal photography and studied animals and how they handled their young. I always marveled at how the mother animal knew how to train a young baby and how she could nurse without ever requiring any classes.

I also noticed that with any animal that I knew, especially the wild animals, the mother always drove off the male when she was getting ready to deliver. She didn't want the male around.

I once said to the husband of a patient who was very much in favor of natural childbirth, "I'm not sure the name natural childbirth fits. If you study nature, you will find that the mother, when she is getting ready to reproduce, always drives off a male so that he is nowhere around. That seems to me to be the natural way."

In a very strident voice, he said to me, "Well, I should hope we are a cut above the animals." So I didn't push my views any further.

I had a patient who was very articulate on this subject. We were discussing whether she would plan to have natural childbirth or not. "I'm certain," she said, "if I absolutely had to, I could go to a dentist and have a tooth out without any Novocain, but as long as he's got Novocain and knows how to use it, I don't see any reason not to choose it."

I liked her reasoning. That was kind of the attitude I took.

Along with the natural childbirth, it became popular among patients to say that they didn't want an episiotomy. An episiotomy is a small incision in the tissue between the vagina and the rectum. The procedure opens the vaginal orifice a little more and allows the baby's head to come out much easier and without the possibility of tearing the tissue. Without the episiotomy, it is frequently impossible for the vaginal opening to stretch enough to allow the baby's head to come through without a tear in the tissue. Sometimes, the lacerations extend all the way into the rectum and quite a repair job has to be done.

It became fashionable among some women to demand that they not have an episiotomy, although one well done is a perfectly clean incision, which heals quickly.

If it is sewed up correctly, it is not particularly painful. There were people who were not well trained who didn't sew them up very well. Some made the medio-lateral episiotomy that went off to the side instead of straight down. The ones straight down divided the tissue in the middle very easily and came back together very easily; there was also much less discomfort. I never could see why women didn't want this to be done and left themselves open to a lot of stretching and tearing. It would have been a longer labor because stretching takes place very slowly. In that day there were some studies showing that continual pressure of the baby's head against this tissue to stretch it out was possibly less than ideal for the baby.

After natural childbirth had reached its zenith, another very good pain reliever for labor came in the form of the epidural. With the epidural, the spinal column was entered with a needle, usually between the third and fourth lumbar vertebrae, which were at the level of the bottom of the spinal cord. We went through the space between the two but stopped before we got into the dura, which covers the spinal cord immersed in fluid. The space is small between the dura and the bony sidewall of the vertebrae. When a pain killer of the Novocain family is injected in that precise location, it spreads outside the dura and anesthetizes the nerves as they emerge from the dura rather than anesthetizing them in the space within the spinal cord. This is safer.

The epidural procedure was somewhat time-consuming, although it wasn't difficult if the needle was placed in the correct location and kept there. The anesthesiologist could do it, and most of the obstetricians could do it, and then the increased use led to having "epidural nurses." Most of the obstetricians had their own epidural nurses. They were trained not only to give the anesthetic but stay with the patients and add more of the anesthesia as necessary through the labor. Part of the technique was to leave a pliable needle in place so that, as the patient's pain increased and as the drug wore off, more could be administered without a new procedure, often for hours at a time. Later, the technique evolved in which a flexible tube was threaded through the needle, and a continuous low-dose medication could be administered throughout labor. This anesthetic method seemed to be very well accepted by most people and seemed to be perfectly safe, an excellent choice for those who did not want natural childbirth. Or the patient could start with natural childbirth and then have the anesthesia for the delivery. Epidural anesthesia is widely used in obstetrics today, and the procedure and administration of medications have undergone many refinements over the years.

Although I thought it was an excellent procedure, I did not do a great many epidurals. This was because by the time these became popular, I had cut down my obstetrical practice and was not taking any patients whom I had not delivered before, which eliminated first babies. Many of my patients who had been brought up on the twilight sleep regimen liked it and just wanted to do that for their last one or two babies.

One of the things which has interested me about the natural childbirth classes is the teaching concerning the importance of immediate bonding between the mother and the baby and the way that would affect the two lives in the future. I conducted a little survey of my own through the years. I was very interested in the women who had adopted babies and then at a later time had conceived and delivered their own. I had a fair number of patients who fell into this category. When they came back to me for checkup, I made a point of asking them what their relationship with the two children was, whether they saw any difference in the two as far as their love for them or their ability to take care of them. Without exception, every single one of them said that they could not tell the difference between the two as far as their emotions toward them, their love toward them or how they treated them.

This made me think that possibly the immediate bonding wasn't as important as it was made out to be. Granted, this was a very unscientific study, and there weren't a great number of people in it, but they were all emphatic. In fact, they usually said that after ten days or so with the adopted baby, they had exactly the same feelings toward it as they did toward their natural child.

FETAL MONITORING

One of the important things that happened late in my career as an obstetrician was the development of the fetal monitor. For years, we relied on telling what was happening with the baby by just listening to the fetal heart through a stethoscope on the mother's abdomen. The normal fetal heart rate was between 120 and 160 beats per minute. If the fetal heart rate got much above that, it was cause to worry and to look out for dangerous things happening. Sometimes during a very prolonged labor, the fetal heart rate would slowly go up and then, as the baby wore out, the fetal heart rate would suddenly drop. The lower fetal heart rates are much more dangerous than the higher ones, but the higher ones let you know that there is a possibility that you are getting into trouble.

However, a fair number of babies would develop fetal heart rates of 180 beats per minute or so with absolutely no problem whatsoever. But under 110, we really began to worry and decide that the baby probably should be delivered fairly shortly. The fetal heart rate frequently would be checked right after a contraction, and if it was low, we would wait and see if it would go back up again to normal. And usually it did. If it didn't, we would begin mentally to explore options for when and how to proceed with delivery.

I remember time and again listening to a fetal heart rate at 60 beats per minute, and my own heart would about stop because I would think every beat is going to be the last, while trying as fast as possible to make preparations for immediate vaginal or cesarean delivery.

The advent of fetal monitors helped the doctor decide what was going on. A fetal monitor is an electronic device that produces a paper print-out, much like an electrocardiogram. It is strapped loosely on the mother's abdomen, positioned over the baby's heart. Clinicians who were well trained in interpretation could tell more about what was going on with the baby than with the stethoscope alone. There were certain signs that warned that even though the fetal heart rate was at a normal rate, the fetus was, in fact, in jeopardy. It could be picked up from the tracing that things were not as they should be or were becoming abnormal.

CESAREAN SECTIONS

The attitude toward cesarean sections has changed markedly. During my training and for some years after that, having to perform a cesarean delivery was almost a defeat. We worked hard to get the patient delivered through the birth canal. This required patience and, often, long labors. At times, we used a technique of resting the patient often, such as by giving her a small dose of morphine. Frequently, the morphine would cause relaxation to the point that the woman would get into good labor and in two or three hours, would deliver successfully without untoward newborn effects. Now, there seems to be little patience with long labors. Obstetrics has gone from a hands-on approach by the obstetrician to a philosophy of either doing nothing or doing a cesarean section. If the patient is not making progress, the doctors go ahead and section her. Another part of the explanation is the fact that sections now are safer than they used to be.

I was never happy about being away from the hospital when the patient was in good labor because the reason the woman has an obstetrician on the case is to act quickly when an emergency comes up. Anybody can deliver a baby if everything is going well. But in times of real crisis, an obstetrician should be right there. I always tried to be there because I was uncomfortable, if I was home, wondering what was going on. I couldn't rest even in the middle of the night.

Infertility Work

I was interested in infertility and did quite a bit of infertility work, but in that situation the physician may never know if what was done really helped or whether the patient would have gotten pregnant anyway. I had patients in my obstetrical practice who had been married 10, 15, even 20 years and had suddenly become pregnant with no fertility work at all, so my interest kind of waned in that. Now, there is some talk of psychotherapy helping infertility. I wouldn't be surprised if that was true. While research has uncovered treatable causes of previously unexplained infertility, we certainly have also seen people who are infertile, have then adopted a baby and have become pregnant without any additional fertility work being done.

One of the cases I will always remember is that of a patient who came to me with infertility, very anxious to have a child. In due time, after only simple interventions, she became pregnant and the pregnancy went along very well with no sign of any difficulties. She went into labor on Christmas morning.

She delivered an anencephalic baby—there was almost no brain. There was little above the level of the spinal cord, no brain or skull above the level of the eyes. The baby lived only a few hours. Everyone involved was very upset. There was, of course, no fault involved. It was before use of ultrasound and before routine administration of folic acid in prenatal vitamins. To this day, on Christmas afternoons, I think about this patient and how her tragedy affected all of us.

Practice of Gynecology

The practice of gynecology is somewhat different from obstetrical practice. Most frequently, a gynecologist is the only doctor a woman has for the years of her life between ages 20 and 60. The gynecologist, pretty much by default, finds himself being a primary care physician for her. The Gyn specialist doesn't necessarily have to take care of the everyday medical problems, but patients often expect it. They will call for a cold or a flu or a gastrointestinal upset. Most gynecologists will treat them and will refer the things outside of his or her expertise.

MEDICAL HISTORY

One thing I always tried to do, which is sadly getting to be old fashioned in some practices, is to take my own histories. I think a history is an extremely valuable thing in making a diagnosis, especially in a difficult case. I know a good many doctors who nowadays let the nurse take the history, or they have some sort of checklist. The advantage of taking the history oneself, and it need not be terribly time consuming, is that an answer will suggest something else, leading off in another more therapeutic direction for the questions. This may sound peculiar, but I would get an idea whether the patient is telling the truth or not. Some patients really don't want to disclose what the main problem is. So many symptoms have a basis in psychology and the emotions of the patient. A good history leads to lots of information that may have nothing to do with the chief complaint. I might learn about the children and what her attitudes are toward them, and what her attitudes are toward her husband and his job or toward a former wife. This used to come up fairly frequently. All of this enters into helping this patient handle her life better.

PHYSICAL EXAMINATION

I felt that every patient who came in, if she hadn't been seen in the very recent past, deserved a thorough physical examination. By that, I don't mean a complete exam, but every woman at every visit (unless the visits are very close together) should have a breast exam. While examining the breasts, the physician might as well take the blood pressure and listen to the heart rate and the lungs. It doesn't take but a minute more. It is advisable when doing a pelvic exam to check the whole abdomen to be sure the liver is not enlarged or that there isn't a mass in the kidney or colon. This always seemed to me to be the role that a doctor should play. In other words, my philosophy was that you are a doctor first and a specialist second. I tried to practice in this way. It is interesting when, in doing so, some things of importance turn up.

I remember several people in whom I found an undiagnosed heart irregularity. It wasn't uncommon for someone to come in with systolic blood pressure over 200 who hadn't been seen by anybody in some time. I would send them to internal medicine specialists and get them taken care of.

Occasionally, while examining a patient, there can be other surprises besides unexpected diagnoses. During a routine physical examination of one of my regular patients, I was performing a breast examination. Fighter planes fly over Asheville from Greenville, South Carolina, and try to fly under the radar up the valleys to Knoxville, Tennessee. Two went over the office that day, flying very low. The building shook. The noise was terrible. As they passed over and got a little bit out of range, I said, "Gee, they're low!"

The patient sat up and said, "They aren't bad when I sit up!"

One of the problems in medicine is the fact that patients aren't paid enough attention as individual people, and some doctors aren't thorough. Too often, they concentrate on one little thing and don't do enough examinations. When a woman comes in complaining about an Ob/Gyn problem, of course the physician is going to do a pelvic exam. But it is important to realize that one in eight hundred have cancer of the breast, and therefore, the breasts should be checked at the same time. That isn't done often enough. Another problem is the dependence on lab work. I use mammograms as an example of relying too much on lab data. I've seen patients who have come to me after they have been told the mammogram was negative, but they had a cancer. Mammograms have up to a 10% false-negative rate. It depends a lot on how good the person is who is reading it. Fortunately, a lot of radiology groups now have someone who is specially trained in mammography interpretation.

Recently, since my retirement, a woman who had been a patient of mine for years called me. I hadn't seen her in over 13 years. She was very upset. In 1987, she'd had a breast removed for cancer. Since that time, she had not had regular checkups, and she had not had regular mammograms. Now she had discovered a fairly sizable lump in her remaining breast, and she couldn't find a doctor who would see her.

In asking her about the situation, I found that several months earlier, she had been in a family practitioner's office. The doctor did not examine her breast and did not ask her if she had a mammogram recently.

The woman who has had cancer in one breast, has a 10% chance of having it in the other breast, so it should very carefully be checked every year. I can't imagine a doctor seeing a patient like that and not examining her and asking her about screening. It really makes me very angry because it is such bad medicine!

As with any technical adjunct in patient care, the mammogram needs to be used properly. There is too often a problem of a patient having a mammogram that is negative and then thinking that there is no chance that she had a cancer. There has been such a push to get every woman to have mammograms and their value has been so extolled; yet it hasn't been equally emphasized to the women and—in some instances—to the doctors that there is a significant number of false negatives.

Once or twice a year, I would examine a breast and find a mass there. Maybe I was sure it was cancer, or maybe I wasn't positive, but if it was a definite mass, I would tell the woman that it had to be biopsied. The patient would often say, "Oh, no. It doesn't need to be."

I would respond, "Why not?"

"Well, I just had a mammogram, and the mammogram was negative."

I would say, "Well, you need to have a biopsy."

And the biopsy would turn out to be cancer.

There is a false sense of security with a negative mammogram. Mammograms are able to pick up very small cancers—so small they cannot be felt—which can be cured readily. But it can miss a few others. My philosophy was, and I am certain that it was the right one, that if there is something in a breast that you can feel, then it has to be biopsied no matter what the mammogram shows.

I can think of two cases where the patients told me—when I discovered a lump—that they had been to doctors whom I considered to be good surgeons, and they had ordered mammograms, and the mammograms had been negative. The physicians had told them they were all right. I insisted on biopsy in each case and the lesions turned out to be cancer. In fact, this problem has been a source of lawsuits on occasion.

Some of the difficulties in medicine today are due to too much dependence on laboratory work. I have told younger doctors, "If the laboratory work does not agree with your clinical idea of a case or the diagnosis, do not sell yourself short. The lab work is very helpful, but when there is a mass in the breast that can be felt and the mammogram doesn't agree, then it is a fairly simple matter to do a biopsy or take out the mass and make a complete diagnosis. If it's negative, fine. But if it is positive, you may have saved your patient's life."

SURGERY

I believe that surgery is a real art form, if the procedure is performed smoothly and with rhythm, as I always tried to do. This concept was introduced to me by Dr. Irving. He was always saying to us in surgery, "Make it an art. Make it an art. Don't plow along through it."

Surgery goes well if it is done gently. Certain orthopedic cases can't be done gently, but abdominal and reparative surgery can be performed very smoothly. It is enhanced by having a good team—an assistant who knows his or her business and a scrub nurse who is used to you.

I hired my own scrub nurse—a woman who operated with me for several years. She was part of my team. Things went smoother that way.

One thing followed another throughout the operation. The next step came in a fluid and rhythmic way. No stopping, hesitating, going back or changing my mind. I felt a real rhythm when things were going right, and the team was working.

One time, I was operating on a very large cancer of the uterus that had filled the whole pelvis. I had to clamp down under it to get it out, but to get down under it, I couldn't see what I was doing. One of the prime rules of surgery is never to clamp and cut where you can't see. There was no way out of this, so I ended up with most of the clamps on sizeable blood vessels. When the tumor was finally out, I started tying them and removing clamps. I picked up one clamp I didn't think was on anything and took it off. It was on the internal iliac artery, which is the main artery on that side of the pelvis! The blood shot way up in the air, almost to the ceiling light. I had in my hand what we call a sponge stick—a long clamp with a sponge wadded up in the end of it that it can be used for getting blood out of the way. Without even thinking, I jammed it down above the point of bleeding on the common iliac artery, which runs in the pelvis along the bone. I just pushed down on that and closed the artery off, and the bleeding stopped. I could then clean it up and see where the cut in the artery was to clamp it and tie it. I didn't stop to think, "What do I do now?" It just happened.

I can still see it. Dr. Ambrose, the first real anesthesiologist in town, was in his usual mode, sitting at the head of the table, reading a newspaper. When the blood spurted up, I saw out of the corner of my eye that his hand shot up and turned the patient's blood transfusion rate up as far as it would go. He never said a word.

Some of my assistants commented that I never got flustered and was always able to react quickly in an emergency. Some of the credit goes to The Professor. Dr. Irving was telling two or three of us residents, one day, "You guys, when you get home and don't have anything to do, you should sit down and think yourself into the worst possible situation you can get into in surgery. Then think how you are going to get out of it, and when it happens, and it eventually will, you won't have to stop and wonder what to do. You can just act."

I used to do that before a difficult operation. I thought ahead of all the things that could go wrong.

I also credit for my calmness in the operating room a lecture I received during my third year of medicine. Mass General had a ward of 50 children with mastoid infection. The lecture was to be on the subject of this very common condition—mastoiditis. I was not particularly interested in nose and throat pathology. In those days before antibiotics, when children got colds, throat infections and ear infections in the winter time, in many instances these traveled into the mastoid sinus. The mastoid is the bone behind the ear. It is part of the skull. Inside that bone is a cavity, the mastoid sinus. The only treatment for mastoiditis was to break into that bone and clean out the cavity and let it drain. Behind the bone was the cavernous sinus. All the blood from the head drains first into that sinus and then into the vena cava—the largest vein in the body—and then goes on to the heart to be re-oxygenated.

The instructor was a young doctor. He described the operation to us. The surgeon would first chip away the exterior bone of the skull to get into the cavity. When the surgeon entered the mastoid sinus, the next task was to scrape the lining of the mastoid bone to get all the infected tissue out and let it drain. The bone between that lining and the cavernous sinus is very thin. One had to stay away from it because it broke open very easily. If the surgeon were to break through, the blood would well up and there is nothing to clamp to stop it. It would be impossible to place sutures in this bone to stabilize the vessels if they were to rupture.

After he described how challenging it was, he made a little quip that I would remember the rest of my surgical days. He said, "If you break into that bone and the blood wells up and you know you are in real trouble, don't say, 'Oh, my God, what have I done?' Say, 'Ah! There it is!'"

In all my future surgery, I used to attempt, if we got into serious trouble, to say, "Ah! There it is!" I found it to have a very calming effect, so I could continue to work and get out of the trouble I was in.

Nowadays, the problem of mastoiditis is almost never seen because of antibiotics early in the game. They keep the mastoid bone from getting infected.

Cancer surgery can be very challenging. It requires much time and skill to get all the malignant tissue out, and now surgeons are doing something, which in my time they never did—operating on metastases. If there is only one metastasis in the liver, they will go in and take that lesion out. That is somewhat successful, but if there is one that is visible there are probably some microscopic ones that will make themselves visible later. However, if there is any chance at all of getting a single one out and curing the patient, for that individual, it is 100% worthwhile.

When I operated on an advanced cancer, I wanted to get everything out that I could see. I remember with two or three patients, a doctor or doctor's assistant coming in to watch the operation and expressing that I was crazy to do such an extensive operation when it seemed it was bound to fail. But the patient was cured. Just one patient cured is worth a mountain of work.

5

PHYSICIAN-PATIENT COMMUNICATION

My advice to medical students is, "Treat the patients as you would like to be treated if you were the patient." Some time ago, I read about a doctor who had a long bout of cancer, which he knew was going to end in his death. He dictated tapes, without anybody knowing it, of what the doctors said and what they had done and how it affected him. He told his wife she was to give them to the doctors after he died. Some of them were not at all complimentary. Some of the things said to him by doctors were very damaging to his emotions. I think that if more physicians treated patients as they would like to be treated, it would be a good thing.

In the teaching of medicine, there should be some lectures on the art of communication. When dealing with patients, it is so important to find out how they are feeling, what is of value to them and what their home situations are. If they have a very serious disease, requiring that the physician convey some bad news, there are ways of doing that without causing unnecessary suffering. I've felt the need for years for some sort of training for doctors on how to talk with a patient and not come across as blunt. It would save a lot of heartaches along the way between the patient and the doctor.

If new doctors completely disregard the psychosomatic part of medicine, they are going to miss the underlying cause of many diagnoses. I think this should be emphasized in medical schools—and to a certain extent, in residencies—even though the residency may not directly relate to psychosomatic medicine.

I have had patients tell me that when a diagnosis of cancer was made there were some doctors who would simply tell them, "Well, you have probably only just so long to live," or, "There is nothing more we can do for you." That is one of the worst things a physician could say. It seems to me that, while the doctor should not give false hope, things could be phrased differently, such as, "This is a very serious situation, and I am going to keep looking into it to try to find new ways to help you. Research may come along before it is too late, and we'll just keep our eyes on this and keep working at it and try some different things." This gives a patient some hope. Students and residents, whatever field they are in, need to learn the art of talking to these people so they don't destroy them.

Doctors can go far in healing the whole person by listening. Physicians are busy; they are human, and they may be thinking about getting behind in their schedule. They may be concerned about a problem with the next patient or may be pondering whether they have done the best thing for the last patient. But if physicians are willing to take the time to listen to their patients, they may find surprising things bearing on the complaints—opening doors to more effective treatment.

Sometimes, the doctor does listen and counsel the whole patient but her family doesn't perceive it. It can be defense mechanisms at play when patients or their family members don't absorb what they are told. I remember a situation, for example, when I had spent almost an hour trying to tell the husband of a patient what a Class III Pap smear amounted to and what I wanted to do to correct this. I explained that a Class III smear shows cells that are not yet cancerous but over a period of time—without treatment—could become cancerous. I even drew pictures showing what was going on with the cells. He was an educated man with an engineering degree. At the end of that time, I said, "Now do you understand exactly what this is?"

He said, "Yes, I think I do. It means three cells are involved."

I know of a doctor who used to spend a lot of time talking to his patients when he told them they needed an operation. He told them what was wrong, what the surgery was going to do and what the results would be. He told me once that he was very discouraged because, just that day, he had spent about an hour explaining to a woman about her need for surgery for a fibroid uterus. He detailed the possible complications if no operation was done and described the procedure in clear and simple terms.

After she left the office, he got a telephone call from her sister saying, "Would you please tell me what is going on? My sister doesn't know a thing about why you are operating on her." The patients can be so upset at the time that they don't absorb what they are told, and then even the thorough, caring physician can be blamed for not talking to them.

I don't know that there is a perfect model to overcome the natural reaction of denial when a patient faces a troubling diagnosis. Each of us is different. What suits one patient doesn't suit another. Several of the larger specialty groups in my community developed systems that seemed to work very well. For instance, a cardiology group employed a very fine woman with a nursing background who was trained by them to talk to the patients, to tell them what a coronary infarction is and what they can expect in the hospital when someone is admitted with a heart attack. Her discussions with the patient and the family took a lot of the fear out of the situation. This has great holistic benefit because fear can do a great deal of damage.

A similar approach was used in our office. Our nurses had been there a long time, and they knew generally what we were telling patients, and they knew about most of the common things we saw in the office. If they saw the patient was upset, they would take her aside and talk to her. That worked quite well. We didn't tell them to do this. It was just something that evolved.

Some patients express a fear of doctors, seeing them as cold and analytical. Certainly, the average doctor has a bit of an ego; I'll admit that. There is too much of the God-like attitude—I know what is good for you. I say so and don't you question it—although there is less of that than there used to be. I think one of the reasons for this was that fifty years ago, back when I first started, we didn't have the treatments we have now. We couldn't do as well for people. But quite likely, if they thought we could do wonders, the benefit that belief would have on their healing—like a placebo effect—could help.

So if kept under control, a doctor's ego is a good thing. Patients pick up on how the caregiver feels. If physicians project that they know what they are doing and that they are going to help the patient, that is going to have a positive effect on the patient. If carried too far, it is not going to help at all.

I think one thing that has affected the doctor-as-God attitude is that the patients are forcing a change. They won't put up with it. A patient now knows he can go for a second opinion, and he has seen so much on television and read so much. He will ask, "What about this?" or "What about that?" and will argue about it. Doctors who have any sense will bend to it and discuss things. I feel that the patient should know what is going on and why, and if there are other treatments available the patient should be apprised of all of them and make the decision regarding what is to be done.

I would tell medical students, "It can be very difficult for a physician to have a patient questioning everything that you propose. If you sense that they don't have confidence in you, they are the hardest people in the world to take care of." I did not hesitate to suggest that a patient might get a second opinion or go to one of the medical schools, if I sensed that the patient didn't have confidence in what I was doing. "You can't do good medicine under those circumstances."

Some doctors are insulted if the patient wants to go for a second opinion or prefers to get care at a large medical center. Some patients have related to me that a doctor refused to send them somewhere, and I would say, "My cure for that is to get a new doctor." My opinion is that what the patient wants should be taken into consideration. If the patient is going to be happier to go to a medical university setting or somewhere else for another opinion, I want them to go because I don't want to try and take care of someone who isn't sure that I am doing the right thing. It is very difficult to treat such people, and it is not good for them either.

A lot has changed with the development of procedures for informed consent. The physician explains to the patient what can go wrong in an operation or what various treatments there are and the advantages of one treatment over another treatment. Then he or she signs consent for it. We don't give patients chemotherapy without them knowing why they are getting it, how they are getting it and how it is going to affect them.

I think that, without question, the patient wants a fairly close relationship with the physician. It has to be on a professional level, of course, but especially cancer patients say that they wish the doctor would give them a hug once in a while when they come into the office. I think that is very good, while it is also true that doctors, especially in cancer work, have to protect themselves from getting too emotionally involved with too many patients. Sometimes the outcomes are not good, and the physicians just can't keep tearing themselves apart all the time. In addition, if they are too close to patients, it could affect judgment as to what ought to be done. They might tend to shy away from doing something painful or disfiguring to patients if they are too emotionally involved.

That's why there is an adage that doctors shouldn't take care of their own families. To a certain extent, it is difficult to take care of close friends for the same reason. Balancing these two conflicting forces—being personally concerned about the patient and not being too emotionally involved—is a matter of judgment. I believe it's also a matter of training and experience. The physician can be friendly with people, show genuine concern and assure them that he or she has their best interests at heart without being too close to them.

As far as lack of warmth on the part of the physician, I think that often depends on the specialty. I could see that at times in oncologists—persons dealing with cancer all of the time. In most cases, I am sure it is a defense mechanism for the doctor. After all, the physician treats a large number of people over a period of time and gets to know them well, and unfortunately, a fair number of them are going to die. If the doctor gets too involved with them emotionally, each one of those deaths is a personal tragedy. Although there are exceptions, most clinicians can stand only just so much of that. In fact, I have known oncologists who, after ten or fifteen years, just stopped . . . and went into another specialty or into research where they didn't have to deal with continuous loss of patients. There are other specialties where this is a factor, but in contrast, obstetrics is, by and large, a pretty happy specialty. The patient is young, she has a self-limiting condition, and, for the most part, she is happy that she is having a baby, and the husband is happy. If the mother-in-law doesn't raise too much Cain, things go along pretty well. I don't think there is a coldness very often in obstetrician/gynecologists. I may be wrong, but I didn't see it.

However, even Ob-Gyn doctors lose patients—some of whom we may have known for quite some time. We had to take the attitude that we did the very best we could and that what happened was out of our power. We knew what we were doing, did good surgery, sent the patients for the right chemotherapy and did everything that could have been done. Sometimes, the patients whom I was afraid I couldn't cure, but did, balanced the ones that I lost. It was a great lift to see somebody get well who we didn't think would. This compensated, to an extent, for some cancer patients I had—one or two I can think of—who just seemed to have everything turn out bad that could. Nothing worked. We would call all over the country to see if anybody had any different ideas, but it would go from bad to worse.

One of the big changes in obstetrics that affects physician-patient communication has come with the advent of large groups of obstetricians practicing together. In those situations, no physician has an individual relationship with any particular patient.

The large-group physicians have definite time assigned to the office seeing prenatal patients, definite time in the hospital and delivery room and definite time to be with their family. When their particular time with a patient is up, another person takes over. The other person may be very well trained but would have no particular bonding with the patient. An individual physician might have seen her two or three times during the prenatal care, and the other physicians might have each seen her two or three times. Everyone has to depend on the records for information.

This is a good thing in one way because the patient knows that her obstetrician is not exhausted from two or three sleepless nights in a row; but on the negative side, it means that the person on duty at delivery may not be up to date on something about the patient that he would know about if he had taken care of her throughout the whole pregnancy.

The sad fact about the large groups is that sometimes patients might not even know the delivering doctor at all. This could have a deleterious effect because the patient would not have established trust in that doctor.

We found that patients whom we had seen every time they came in the office were more at ease when they were in labor. I suspect that being unfamiliar with the doctor might have something to do with the increase in malpractice cases. I have observed through the years that doctors who did not have good rapport with their patients were much more apt to be sued—whether the suit was justified or not—than the person in whom the patient had great confidence.

I would advise physician trainees to think before speaking. I have occasionally said some things to patients, and the moment the words were out of my mouth, I said to myself, My God, why did I say that? I would advise young physicians to try to remember that what you say and how you say it is going to be perceived by a patient who is afraid and may be in pain. There are often two ways to say the same thing. My advice is, "Treat the patients as you would like to be treated if you were the patient." I have often said that if all doctors had to have a barium enema, there would be fewer barium enemas ordered.

Some time ago, I read about a doctor who had a long bout of cancer, which he knew was going to end in his death. He dictated tapes, without anybody knowing it, of what the doctors said and what they had done and how it affected him. He told his wife she was to give them to the doctors after he died. Some of them were not at all complimentary. Some of the things said to him by doctors were very damaging to his emotions. I think that if more physicians treated patients as they would like to be treated, it would be a good thing.

6

LIFE AFTER CANCER

> I remember one man in his 70s who came in with far-advanced lung cancer. He looked so sick. I wasn't sure he was going to live to get home. Part of that, it turns out, was because he had been told he had a month to live. We encouraged him to get more active. This was in March. He had always been a great gardener, but he was so weak he couldn't get out to do any gardening. He started going out and just sitting on a rock, then he started scratching in the soil, and by June, he had a garden planted. He lived for four years after that, a very active life. He was desperately ill when he came in, but I think just the fact that we convinced him that he wasn't at death's door and that we encouraged him to do things he liked to do put some meaning back into his life. This enabled him to live much longer than he would have. This type of success encouraged us and made us think that the time we were spending was worthwhile.

In medical school, I was very interested in cancer as a disease. When I had an elective month, I took it in cancer pathology. In 1939, when I took my New York State boards at the end of my Boston medical school days, I received a notice that I hadn't passed pathology. I had heard that they "fussed up" guys from good out-of-state-schools. If the student had only one subject area he had failed, he could write in to request that he would not have to take the whole exam over. I contacted the board and said it had been my best subspecialty course in medical school and I didn't understand why I had failed. The letter I received back said they reexamined my pathology examination and they passed me.

I studied pathology under Shields Warren, who was one of the country's leading cancer pathologists. I enjoyed that tremendously. He saw some patients along with his pathology work and had quite a lot of good thoughts about treating cancer patients and about their emotions. I always remember him saying, "I have seen a tremendous number of cancer patients in my medical lifetime, and I have never seen a patient who didn't want to live another day." I've since watched that and I tend to agree with him. It is the relatives, a lot of times, who want the family member put out of his or her misery. Of course, there are many diseases that can be worse as terminal illnesses than cancer. An example is amyotrophic lateral sclerosis (ALS)—Lou Gehrig's disease. I can see that as a very difficult cross to bear.

With the increasing interest in euthanasia—there is quite a lot of talk in some of the European countries like Denmark and Holland—I have had to think about it from a doctor's standpoint. I've come to the conclusion that I personally would not be able to perform it. I would not be upset with someone else if they thought they could, especially if there were safeguards, such as a panel of doctors reviewing the case. One of the problems I see with some of the euthanasia procedures that have been done in the States is that they have been done way too early. It seems premature to perform it almost at the time of diagnosis of a disease, even though it is expected eventually to become terminal. I think from a practical standpoint, that is not good.

There is so much research being done now, and so much is coming out on some of these diseases, that there might be a cure before long. New things are being developed all the time. We've seen it over and over in cancer work—something which looked very grim, six months later might have close to a 100% cure rate. I think one has to be exceedingly cautious about choosing to end a life.

Every cancer is different from the next one. Of course, each is really a different disease. Cancer of the breast is entirely different from cancer of the cervix or cancer of the stomach. The means to establish the diagnosis for each are different, and each is treated differently.

When results of cancer treatment are good, it's about as satisfying a thing as I know. One of the happiest things to experience is suddenly to run into a patient that I operated on for cancer some 30 years ago and see that she is fine. With so much of medical treatment, I don't really know how much good I've done a patient. Certainly, if I operate on a cancer and the patient lives on and on, I know I've done some good.

Through the years, I became more and more interested in how the mind affected disease. I had seen so many cancer patients either live longer or shorter lives than one thought they should because of an impelling situation. A woman, for instance, who by all medical criteria couldn't live any longer, but who wanted to see a grandchild graduate from college or a grandchild be born or a daughter married or something like that, lived until she saw what she wanted and then died. It seemed obvious to me the emotions had something to do with it.

There is interesting research now showing how the mind affects the body and the body, the mind. Rather than mind-body, I would consider emotions-body as the way of describing it. It is fascinating.

In trying to cure somebody, I want to have everything possible working for me. It is a goal to use all the scientific medicine available. Above and beyond the science, the mind and emotions can affect the cure—make the disease worse or help heal it. In trying to cure somebody of a difficult disease, it is wise to take into consideration their emotions and try to get them to really want to be cured.

MIND-BODY CONNECTION

My interest in the mind-body effect started by observing my aunt, seeing her working on the emotions and spirituality of our family and acquaintances. She felt that there could be an extra-sensory type of communication between people that might be used for healing if it were nurtured. She felt that she had developed such skills and by relaxation and concentration could help people, even at distances. I have no scientific proof that she did any good, but certainly she conquered quite a number of things in herself. She had a bad heart. She did a great deal to help her own condition by her relaxation techniques.

My mother was at the opposite end of the spectrum from my aunt. Her bouts of sickness affected the whole family. I saw what was going on. I was one in the family who realized that her mind was her main problem.

Through my years of practice, I saw that certain people—expected by medical criteria to die very soon—

would live far longer than predicted, as though by just plain refusing to die when they should have. I observed it, especially in cancer patients—and kept it in the back of my mind. I couldn't help but wonder what was going on.

I think that real holistic care means paying attention to the whole person, not concentrating on whatever they say about their complaints. It means doing more than just the scientific part of medicine. It means having the knowledge that disease can be a product of the whole person, not just an appendix or a piece of bowel. Better results come from trying to design the therapy so that good things for general health are included—such as a good diet and exercise.

The family doctor in earlier days did quite a bit of holistic-type medicine. In a sense, that was about all he had to work with. He did not have the knowledge and ability to effect cures like we have today, not because he was dumb, but because the knowledge had not been accumulated for him. There just wasn't much treatment of a lot of diseases before antibiotics and modern surgery.

As science advanced, I don't think there was initially the holistic push that there is today. Even now, there is not a great holistic push among doctors. However, the patients are insisting on it today. Many of the younger doctors who are coming out in family practice are much more holistic. Some of the medical schools are starting courses and departments of alternative medicine, which are bringing in the holistic part of medicine. One could expect in the future, as those students become residents, they would have more grounding in that area.

So many doctors, especially the ones who are middle-aged now, come from extremely scientific medical training with a great emphasis on laboratory work. Unless they are attuned, as some are, to the patient as a whole, along with the scientific part of it, they are just not going to be holistically inclined. The journals they read are all about new techniques of surgery or new combinations of chemotherapy. Drugs are coming out at a terrific rate. Keeping up with all that can be very time-consuming. In a busy practice, the physician doesn't have time to consider other treatments.

The patients essentially handle the emotional side of the disease by themselves. Some people can do that and some can't. Some are helped by relatives and some are greatly harmed by relatives and neighbors. It has been pretty much up to the patient to find his or her own way emotionally through the disease.

There are cases where the mind has very little to do with disease. If one inherits Huntington's chorea, he is going to have Huntington's chorea. Mind has nothing to do with that. On the other hand, there are diseases that we have known for years, long before all the studies that exist now on mind-body, that are stress-related. People are driven to do some things—work too hard, play too hard, smoke too much. Those and other stressors cause diseases that can be traced back to the mind.

If the immune system is strong, we can ward off the common cold, but if the immune system is depressed, often due to various emotional situations and stress, then, in a second-hand way, disease that ensues is of the mind. We know that emotional changes make the immune system more susceptible to diseases, even to the point of being more susceptible to cancer.

When I first learned about the immune system in medical school, it was purely in the sense of bacteriology and virology and the work that was being done in that. Jenner was one of the early ones to devise vaccines for smallpox. Subsequent work was done by Pasteur without understanding why the vaccination kept people from having the disease. Pasteur proceeded to make other vaccines, such as the rabies vaccine. In my childhood, diphtheria was a big thing. But by medical school, I saw only one case of diphtheria. After my training, the Salk vaccine for poliomyelitis was introduced. But I didn't learn in those training and early practice years about the body's own immune system healing diseases not considered infections, per se.

I don't know how much the mind can affect the infectious type of immunity, but we've known for a long time that people do not get sore throats as much if they keep themselves in good condition.

The first research I know regarding the mind effect on the immune system, was in the study of cancer. Investigators saw that emotions had something to do with how people with cancer fared.

This was not new information. Galen in 200 A.D. wrote that cancer seemed to be a disease of the depressed. And Seneca, a Greek physician about the time of Christ, wrote that part of the cure is the desire to be cured. In the Old Testament book Proverbs, the verse 17:22 says, "A merry heart is good medicine. A downcast spirit drieth the bones." So, way back 600-700 years before Christ, it was noted that emotions had something to do with sickness.

In the late 1950s and early 1960s, the concept resurfaced as we realized that how the individual handled stress, anxiety and depression had something to do with how people handled cancer. In the early 1960s, researchers took rats and divided the litters at birth and raised half of them in a stressful environment and half in a non-stressful environment. Only 10% of the non-stressed rats developed cancer, whereas 90% of the stressed rats incurred the disease. More and more studies along this line followed. In the early-to-mid-1970s, a fair amount of research was published—good research, controlled research—showing that the emotions did seem to affect outcomes, having a great deal to do with how the immune system functions. We had known for a long time that there was an immune system against bacterial infections and diseases, but now researchers found there was an immune system against malignant cells and that certain defenses of the body and blood would kill cancer cells.

We know now that we all make cancer cells, all through our lives. If this immune system is functioning correctly and if there are not too many cancer cells at one time, the immune system destroys them as they are made and a clinical cancer does not develop. This is much the same as people who have a positive tuberculin test, but they have never had tuberculosis that they know of. They have just taken in a few bacilli in their lifetimes, and the immune system killed them off before they got the disease. If the immune system had been down because of emotions or stress, or because the body was tired—if they were in a concentration camp, for example—they probably would have gone on and died of the disease.

I think people who do meditation and relaxation get both physical and emotional benefit. The relaxation allows the body to function better and apparently also affects hormone balance, circulation, and, quite likely, the brain chemistry. Endorphins, which can benefit the immune system, are affected by relaxation and meditation techniques.

In the 1970s, Texans O. Carl Simonton and Stephanie Matthews-Simonton published in medical journals and in a classic best-selling book, *Getting Well Again*, that therapeutic-emotional intervention seemed to be prolonging lives of some cancer patients and that cancer patients did better if they had help with the psychological part of the disease. Studies showed that, in people under stress, the immune system function diminished.

A patient of mine with breast cancer got some tapes of the Simonton Method and gave them to me. I went over them and was very interested in them. I wasn't 100% convinced, but it piqued my interest in an area that already held fascination for me. I asked one of the local counselors, Don Boone, who is very good in his profession, to listen to the tapes and see what he thought. Afterward, we met and discussed it and decided that it wouldn't hurt to try it. That is how we started Asheville's program of Life After Cancer in 1977.

LIFE AFTER CANCER

The program was pretty innovative at the time and was only the third one in the country, as far as we could tell.

We began to get good results with cancer patients. We helped them a lot with the side effects of chemotherapy. At that time, some of the patients had been starting to vomit when they turned into the drive at the chemotherapist's office, expecting to be sick. We met at my office on Saturdays. On the floor below were the only two oncologists in town at the time. We went down and talked to them about it, and their nurses started referring patients up to us. Some patients in the group became easier to treat because they weren't having as many symptoms from the chemotherapy. They were handling the emotional side of everything better. Doctors were interested because it made their work less troublesome, so they referred more patients to us. We soon had two or three patients who did so much better that it encouraged us greatly.

I remember one man in his 70s who came in with far-advanced lung cancer. He looked so sick. I wasn't sure he was going to live to get home. Part of that, it turns out, was because he had been told he had a month to live. We encouraged him to get more active. This was in March. He had always been a great gardener, but he was so weak that he couldn't get out to do any gardening. We encouraged him first to start just walking out to his garden and sitting on a rock and looking at it. Then he started scratching in the soil, and by June, he had a garden planted. He lived for four years after that, a very active life. He was desperately ill when he came in, but I think just the fact that we convinced him that he wasn't at death's door and the fact that we encouraged him to do things he liked to do put some meaning back into his life. This enabled him to live much longer than he would have without it. This type of success encouraged us and made us think that the time we were spending was worthwhile.

The format of the Life After Cancer work was not complicated. I would take the new patients and explain to them what the research was and how it could be helpful. I was very careful not to tell anyone that we were going to cure them, or even that we were going to make them any better. I explained what the research showed and tried to put the idea across that what time they had left, they ought to spend living and not just sitting, waiting for something to happen. One of the ideas we used was derived from the work of Dr. Lawrence LeShan in New York, a prolific researcher who was very prominent in this field. He used to say, "It's not adding years to your life that counts, but adding life to your years."

We encouraged patients to add life to whatever time they had, whether it was a month or ten years. We stressed that we were not curing anybody and would not take anybody into the group who was not going on with their medical therapy. Don Boone was continuing to work with me. His background was in psychiatric social work, and he was very competent at therapy. He was able to do some remarkable things in turning people's emotions around to a positive attitude.

We did a lot of work with relaxation techniques that had been proven by laboratory work to be very useful. Besides relaxation, we used visual imagery, a technique that has since been found to be of value. The patient was instructed to visualize being well. We did a lot of work with self-esteem. Patients did much better with an improved self-image. Some people thought that the cancer reduced their self-esteem. If they were diseased, in those days, more than now, there was the thought that there was some sin they had committed and this was God's retribution. In fact, I could hardly contain myself once in the hospital when I heard a minister praying beside a patient for God to remove the sin from her that had caused the disease. We had to cope with concepts like that in the Life After Cancer group.

We did the relaxation techniques in groups. We would present them as a teaching process and encourage the patients to do them at home. We would enlist one of the patients to lead the group once he got so he could. Some of them were very, very good at it. This was also helpful for the families who came, husbands with their wives or wives with their husbands. I remember one patient who lived in Knoxville who was too sick to come. Her daughter, who was taking care of her, used to come each Saturday from Knoxville and attend the group and take what she learned back to the patient. We occasionally had individuals attend who had a great deal of malignancy in the family and were thus probably genetically predisposed toward cancer. Free of malignancy at the time, they would try to do what we were teaching as a preventative measure for the disease.

If the original premise of Life After Cancer were to be expanded, an ideal mind-body center might go in two directions. One would be to get more people with cancer to accept the fact that this could be a help to them—not a cure, but a great help—in living a full life and also a great help for their families. A group evolved in our program for families to attend. That included not only group therapy and individual therapy, but also diet and exercise, emphasizing the importance of the latter in and of themselves.

We have to work harder to convince people that they have to do this to help themselves. Too many people are passive, do what the doctor tells them and hope for the best. They don't think about changing their lifestyle. People who have been at Life After Cancer who have done the best—and some of them have added years of good living to their lives—have changed lifestyles. I must say that most of them have died better deaths than the average person. Many of our people have lived active and productive lives with their disease and then, within just a week, have gone downhill and died instead of experiencing a long, prolonged illness. Sometimes, it seemed as though they simply decided that the time had come.

The second direction that an ideal center would take is preventative, getting on a good diet and a healthy lifestyle, using exercise and relaxation techniques when there is no cancer. This has been worked on a great deal at Harvard. Dr. Benson, who is a Professor of Medicine at Harvard Medical School, has studied this for twenty years. His sphere of interest was hypertension and diabetes. He is a great believer that people who take time to do relaxation and meditation have fewer diseases and live longer than those who rush on through the hustle and bustle of life. Benson was a great believer in people with some spiritual aspect of their lives doing better.

Preventive health care is an important component of life after cancer. If the patients are doing all those healthy things like diet, exercise and relaxation, I think they have a proper mindset; they have taken some responsibility for themselves. That is very important. So many people who have cancer are passive; they want the doctors to cure them, and if they can't, well, tough luck. By contrast, with preventive care, instead of getting sick and expecting people to fix them, they are demonstrating personal responsibility.

My interest in emotions and cancer and starting Life After Cancer presented some problems. This was not a view held by very many, in spite of the fact that there was some good research to show that it had a scientific background. As we started the group, I was not one to go out, get on the stump and try to get believers, and perhaps did not push what we were doing as hard as I might have. I just didn't want to make an appeal to people on an emotional basis. I wanted to have scientific proof for what we were doing.

I wanted to convince people that it was worthwhile because there was good scientific research to show that the emotions did have something to do with how people got along with the disease and the course the disease took. We did some explaining to medical society meetings and wrote a paper about our experiences, which a major journal in obstetrics and gynecology rejected for publication, saying it was not scientific. Mostly, we let the patients who were helped advertise for us. The cancer patients could show, in many instances, that they could alter the course of the disease by altering their emotions and leading a healthier life in general—especially a healthier emotional life.

I presented a paper at the South Atlantic Association of Ob/Gyn annual meeting about our experiences with this and cited the research on which it was based. The organization covers all the Southeastern states from Maryland to Florida, including Texas. The report received good reviews and particular support from an investigator with similar experiences at the University of Miami. He had statistics to show that patients in his hospital who were exposed to this philosophy only during the time that they were in-patients after the cancer surgery stayed in the hospital a shorter period of time, had less pain medication and went back to work faster after they were discharged. One of the discussants of the paper, who got up after I had given the report, stated that this was probably the most important paper of the four-day meeting. On the other hand, some of the other discussants didn't see any value in it. Doctors reacted in various ways, and I just accepted the fact that it wouldn't appeal to everyone. A Medical University of South Carolina academician predicted this concept would become widely accepted in the future.

We gained a great deal of support from the nurses of oncology patients. They noted that their patients on chemotherapy would have far fewer side effects that could be attributed to emotions if they received intervention at the Life After Cancer program. The nurses observed that some patients who came for their weekly intravenous treatments would start vomiting when they turned into the driveway to the office. That happened much less often in our patients.

Some of the patients went to various medical schools to participate in research chemotherapy protocols. The new drugs being studied often had far more numerous side effects. The patients came back and reported that the doctors at the centers didn't understand why they had fewer side effects than the general population who were coming to them.

Some people came to Life After Cancer because they knew that their friends or relatives had benefited from it; others chose not to come because they told us they didn't want to be associated with a bunch of other patients who were very sick. However, some of the people who came told us they were amazed to see that, to their surprise, our patients didn't seem to be in bad shape. They had expected on their first visit to see a room full of very sick, dying patients, but there were people laughing and chatting and seeming perfectly normal. This impressed them a great deal.

It was interesting that some of the doctors who referred us patients didn't refer all their patients. It was sometimes obvious that a patient was referred to us because they were difficult for the doctor to handle and he was tired of trying to deal with all of their psychological problems.

Although some of the patients didn't take to the program and did not improve, it was very gratifying for us to see that some of the people were really being helped. Don Boone, who started this with me, was a superb counselor—highly trained. He had a way of getting the people to change their lives and start coming out with the best that was in them.

We had quite a few people who were very sick when they first came. In fact, I think of two people who had been told they only had a month to live. They were literally sitting and waiting to die. With Don's help and inspiration, they started to live productive lives.

A woman, who was highly intelligent with a fine education, had been told she had a month to live. After attending our program, she got interested in survival and led a productive and interesting life. She entered into her daughter's hobby of rifle-shooting marksmanship, went around with her daughter to international shooting exhibitions and was an official at some of them. She lived more than four years. I'm convinced that she would have lived longer than one month without any intervention, but she surely would not have lived as satisfying a life if she had not been encouraged.

We saw patients with cancer who, in spite of how long they were told they were going to live, wanted to live to see a certain event take place, such as a daughter getting married or a grandchild being born or somebody graduating from college. They far outlived the expectations of their doctors to see this event happen. Of course, we encouraged this type of thing as much as we could.

The time we spent—all of which was free time away from our families on Saturday mornings—was very satisfying. It was very rewarding to us to see these people live longer than expected and live productive, meaningful lives.

One of the things that bothered us, and still does, is that so many people refused to take advantage of this help that was available to them—mostly because their doctors were not particularly interested in it. Now, more are. The younger doctors who are coming out of medical school have had more exposure to alternative types of medicine and the knowledge of the emotions and its effect on various diseases.

The methodology that the Life After Cancer groups used was to challenge people to change their lives. Patients were shown, in some instances at least, that they were not doing the best for themselves with their particular lifestyles. One of the common problems was that the patient did not stick up for himself or herself in life. They were almost doormats with other people getting them to do this, that or the other thing instead of doing what they wanted to do themselves—especially in family life. Don and I often thought that one of the problems with many of them was that they had been brought up under the guise of "love thy neighbor as thyself", but forgot the "as thyself" part. They sacrificed themselves to do whatever they could for other people. We agreed with the observations of the researchers that this was pretty bad for them emotionally and psychologically.

Our groups were set up, not as support groups entirely, but as support-therapy groups. To get anything out of the groups, patients had to enter into the therapy of their own emotions and change their own lives. Thinking back on the patients I have seen do so well, most of them made major changes in their way of living. Sometimes the changes didn't suit their families because the family was used to having "mother do everything for them." When mother suddenly said that she wanted to do so and so for herself, that upset the family equilibrium considerably, but it did mother a lot of good when she learned to do this.

We have been associated with quite a few support groups starting up. Churches would call and ask us to come out, talk to members and get them started. Those groups never seemed to last very long. Sometimes, they would be referred to as "pity parties" because everybody commiserated with each other without doing anything to change their lifestyle situations.

The Life After Cancer groups gradually grew until we were having two groups on Saturday morning of twenty-five to thirty people. These were just too big to do much therapy. As our groups got bigger, we had to have more help, and we were fortunate to have several volunteers who were trained therapists like Don. Some of them have stayed with us for many years. We were greatly indebted to them. They picked up many valuable ways of running groups from Don. They were very loyal to us—giving up Saturday mornings for no pay. They—like the rest of us—really believed in what we were doing.

I was invited to Atlanta to speak at a large cancer conference and share our results and some of the research involved. Part of the program was a panel of five fairly youngish people, all of whom had far advanced cancer, who were expected to die in a reasonably short period of time, and who had essentially finished their treatment.They all told their stories. Each one of them had made a major turnaround in his or her lifestyle—either rid themselves of a marriage which was pulling them down, or changed jobs they didn't like for something they did like, or other drastic moves. Each one of these five people was at the time of the panel free of disease when they had been thought to be dying of it. Each one of them had made a very major change in their lifestyle before the cancer began to get better.

One of the things I want to point out is that we do not and never have claimed that these therapy support groups will cure cancer. I don't claim cures for the people who have done so well when they were expected to do poorly. I think what happens is that they allow the body to bring forth its natural healing powers. I would not for a minute promise anybody that going to groups like this was going to cure them, or even that it was going to extend their life expectancy. However, at the very least, almost all of them that really enter into it will have a much better life for the time that they live than they would without the help of the group.

As we progressed in Life After Cancer in the early 80s, we had more and more people coming and were obviously helping some of them; this was one reason for continuing to work with it. It was very fulfilling to see people begin to live again after being pushed down with the emotion and fear of the diagnosis of cancer. Some of them were literally sitting down and waiting to die when they still had good years ahead of them.

Then, as Life After Cancer got bigger and bigger, we began to develop problems. Mostly, we got bigger because of patients telling other patients. We didn't get bigger because of referrals from the doctors. Only the occasional doctors would buy into what we were doing. Physicians were not the least bit antagonistic to us—we were not a threat—but they didn't really think it was worth spending their time to talk people into coming. People frequently had to be convinced that it was worthwhile, and that took time. They just resisted. Society resisted it. So we didn't have much help from the doctors.

Now this form of intervention is fairly common. In those days, it was brand new and, to some, it smacked a little bit of witchcraft. Doctors were trained, and still are, in science. Anything that didn't show up on an X-ray or in lab work or that didn't lend itself to controlled studies was just not worthy of their interest. They didn't take the time to read the literature despite the supportive evidence in good scientific articles.

The average doctor has a great deal of difficulty keeping up with anywhere near the amount of literature that is poured out—given the amount of studies and research that are published in any one phase of medicine. Until the medical schools and the residency programs begin to teach the effect of the emotions on cancer and create solid research on the subject, it will be very difficult to get the average doctor to become interested in this.

I think that one of the reasons some oncologists shy away from this type of thing is a matter of self-protection. Oncology is a very difficult specialty psychologically for the individual who is practicing. The cancer subspecialist has so many people who do not get along well. Some physicians believe they would not be able to withstand psychologically the emotional effects of a continual number of patents who do not get along well, if they were to get too involved with them. The natural tendency is to keep them on a very scientific level, expressing interest in the progress and in new things coming out that might increase the survival percentages and decrease the side effects, but not getting involved on a very personal level. The end result staves off the bitter disappointment when things do not work.

Therefore, one of the challenges that was associated with the growth of Life After Cancer was finding the right professionals to work with us in the group. We couldn't take just any trained counselor or psychologist to work in this atmosphere. One would think that there would be plenty of psychologists or psychiatrists who were interested in this. Unfortunately, even some of the few we had did not pan out. They couldn't get into what we were doing well enough to be of help. That limited our growth because, in a situation like this, the actual persons running the groups are the ones who make or break the group. They either attract the people to continue or they detract from the organization.

The board lapsed into not working hard. I did a lot of speaking to promote support when I was invited to do so and tried to find additional places to speak. People liked what they heard but they didn't jump on the band wagon in any great numbers or come through when we began to need money after our expansion. United Way did not contribute anything even though I felt they were giving an inordinate amount of money to some of the organizations in town that were not doing anywhere near the amount of good that we were. Now, as I look back on it, I wonder whether I was a little bit afraid, subconsciously at least, of pushing the organization too much. I really don't know why that would have been, unless it was my personality. There was kind of a feeling that I didn't want to make waves. I certainly did not get out and work as hard as I might have. But at the same time, I had a busy practice.

One of the things that I am probably most proud of in my career occurred toward the end of my years in medicine. I was given the Outstanding Physician Award in 1979 by the Buncombe County Medical Society. This was an award that is not given every year. In fact, I think there have only been about nine of them awarded in the history of the society, which goes far back. I was very proud to have my peers vote this for me. One of the things which the president of the society emphasized, when making an introductory speech, was the fact that I had, for some years, given my free time on Saturday mornings working to get Life After Cancer started and to carrying it forward. The award meant a great deal to me, and still does because, as I've said before, I always wanted to be the best medical doctor I could and practice the best medicine I could. Apparently, I impressed other people and my peers that I was doing that. I don't know if this negates the idea that they weren't supportive.

In my gynecology practice, I came to realize after some years that many of the complaints for which women came to me were essentially caused by tension and their environment. I sometimes felt that I was not doing them justice as I tried to help them. I really wished I had the help of a well-trained counselor. They kept coming back, again and again, with the same type of complaints that it seemed obvious to me, were psychosomatic—nothing would help them. So, I finally convinced my partners that we should take on a trained counselor to assist in some of these cases which were such a problem. It didn't work out as I hoped it would. She soon got so busy she didn't have time to take new people whom we wanted to refer to her, or to see somebody who was really in crisis while in the office. She wouldn't be able to drop her other appointments to see her. Actually, after a couple of years, we had to terminate her because the company with whom we had our malpractice insurance told us that they couldn't insure us if she was there. She had her own malpractice insurance from her association. They said correctly that if she got sued, we would be sued too, since she was our employee. They would not be responsible for any malpractice suits brought against us for anything she might have done. So she went out on her own.

If a new group were to start, it seems to me that it ought to be enough to explain to the community what is behind the care scientifically—why there is reason to intervene. The next step would be to share some of the results. That may not be enough but it is about all the advice I am able to give.

The key to success of a new group would be a well-trained, charismatic leader like Don Boone who believed in the basic tenets. The patients received significant help from his methods in the group therapy, wanted to come back and wanted to get other people to come. When he got so busy in his own practice that he could no longer do the Life After Cancer work, we never quite replaced him.

I feel good about having brought Life After Cancer to Asheville and having developed it to the position at which it is now, although it is still not accepted in a large part by the medical community. I feel that because of the interest of the younger doctors and the medical school teaching of the value of this care, the concept will stay and grow. This organization, or one with the same concept, will eventually prosper and become a big part of the medical/therapeutic community.

I think of one person who lives 20 or 30 miles away from here who came into our group. She was dedicated to doing everything her daughter and husband wanted her to do. She had a far-advanced cancer, but it was not hopeless. Finally, after quite a few sessions, she came in very happy one Saturday morning to the group, just bubbling over, and seemed to have a complete change. We asked her what was going on and she said, "Well, this morning I got up and, after breakfast, I said I was going to Life After Cancer. My husband said he wanted the car to do something, and my daughter said she wanted to go somewhere and I would have to take her there. I simply declared that I was going to Life After Cancer and got into the car and drove away."

This change of attitude is one of the things we've witnessed when people are very successful. There are others—major things. Somebody who has been living with a spouse and hating every minute of it for years will suddenly come to the realization that this isn't the way to live, and they will break up—and the patient is much better for it. We obviously don't try to get them to break up. We try to get them to straighten the whole thing out.

This is an example of what we confront. It has to be done to do the patients any good. I remember a woman in a town nearby who was all upset and tensed up over the fact that she had a swimming pool in the yard, and in the summer all the neighborhood kids came and swam in the swimming pool. The children would keep running in and out of her house to go to the bathroom and would keep dripping water in the living room and kept the bathroom reasonably dirty. It was quite a problem to get her to put her foot down and finally get rid of all this tension she was living under.

Years ago, before there was any help in this way for patients, I did a mastectomy on a very beautiful, 35-year-old woman. Despite extensive preoperative counseling, when she woke up with her breast gone, she just sank into the deepest of depressions. For two days, I tried to talk with her and didn't get anywhere. She was just too depressed over what she thought her looks were going to be. I had an inspiration. I called a patient who was about her age, a very good-looking, vivacious woman on whom I had performed a similar operation two or three years before, and whom I knew well socially. I said to her, "You've got to help me." I told her about this young woman and said she should go in and talk with her. She was leading an extremely active life. Without further promoting, she put on a short tennis dress—low-cut in the front—tucked a tennis racket under her arm and bounced in to talk to her. The next time I went in to see the patient, there was a 180-degree change. She was up and ready to go and everything was fine.

That was before the days of Reach to Recovery, a program that I applaud which is run by the American Cancer Society. It has done so much good in similar ways for breast cancer patients. A group of women who had mastectomies underwent some training provided by the American Cancer Society. With their doctor's permission, they called on individuals in the hospital who had just had a mastectomy. The patient saw that here was a woman who was healthy and well and looked okay. The Reach to Recovery person told them about problems they might have and told them about exercises for the arm and where to get a prosthesis and what kind of prosthesis is best. It has been a very great help to mastectomy patients through the years. I am 100% behind it.

I've found that a great concern of mastectomy patients is how this will affect their husbands. So I did a little study on my own, asking husbands about their views after their wives had mastectomies. Without exception, the husbands said it made absolutely no difference to them. Usually, I got the comment, "I didn't marry a breast, I married her." This is a thing that most married mastectomy patients do ponder, I know. For some of them, it is a major thing in deciding whether to have a mastectomy or not. But, from my short study in talking to husbands, it is not a problem as far as husbands are concerned.

The question of the survival of groups like Life After Cancer is a matter of considerable concern to people interested in this type of intervention and one to which I have given considerable thought. I think that one of the problems facing such groups is the fact that medicine has evolved into a business—a business that must show a profit. Medicine has been taken over in all sorts of business ways, much to its detriment.

As I think about what would be ideal in medical treatment now, both for the patient and the doctor, it seems to me that we have to change our ideas considerably. In dealing with cancer patients, we guide them in how to react to disease and how they could strengthen their immune systems. In order for their bodies to be able effectively to combat the disease to the best of their ability, we have to get most of them to change their attitude about life and lifestyle. I think that to have a more perfect delivery of medical systems than we have now—to engender more acceptance by the patients, we physicians also have to change our whole attitude toward it.

SPIRITUALITY AND HEALTH

There is a lot of research that shows a spiritual person does much better in fending off disease, conquering it and staying healthy than a non-spiritual individual. There is something there that we don't understand. Most of us seem to need something spiritual to hang onto, and I can't define this particularly. It is something that is sensed. To me, it is still one of the unexplained things. It seems to me that there is some sort of a source of strength out there. We have a lot more power than we ever use. In World War II, I heard that out in the Pacific, in the bombing of a carrier, a bomb landed in the middle of the deck and didn't explode. It was a 250-pound bomb, yet one of the guys was able to pick it up and dump it over the side. We hear sometimes of a car tipping over and trapping somebody, and of rescuers using strength that they never thought they had to lift the car off the person trapped beneath it.

I see an analogy in sports. I like to watch athletics. You see, time and again, an athlete or a team that is very good, and the next week someone scores on them early, they go to pieces, and the whole thing falls apart. It's another indication of the mind-body situation.

The connotation of spirituality may be completely misunderstood. There are certain types of things that are routinely called spirituality—especially in the Christian religion—that are not healthy. What we see frequently in cancer patients is that they take the teaching of the church—that you should love your neighbor as yourself—too literally. They have worked that around in their lives to the place where they spend all their time helping others and give no thought to themselves. Of course, you can't love others effectively unless you love yourself and help yourself.

In medical school teaching, educators are now beginning to emphasize this. By spirituality, I do not mean any particular religion but a sense of the spirit. Spirituality is a lifestyle that admits to a larger force in the universe. It may not be a controlling force, but one that can be used as a guide for living. To me, the basis of spirituality is a feeling of love and consideration for yourself and others, for the world and the environment. I think it is an admission that there is something outside of ourselves, outside of the animal part of us, which helps us through life and helps to control our actions and our thoughts and gives us a sense of values. It's a hard thing to describe.

It is pretty well accepted now among people who are doing studies in this area that a sense of spirituality does help healing. There have been actual laboratory studies that show that people who are spiritual—who pray or meditate regularly—have fewer diseases and do better with treatment than people who apparently have no thought of any outside spirit or guide. Today, among a great many doctors and researchers, it is a foregone conclusion that a sense of spirituality does help ward off disease and heal the person who is sick. This doesn't mean that people who are spiritual don't get sick and die—they certainly do. Dr. Benson, professor of medicine at Harvard, has performed research in this area for many years. He states that spirituality is almost a necessity in curing many diseases. Dr. LeShan has said, "No patient will be permanently cured of cancer without a spiritual base in their living."

Studies show that people who are members of close-knit groups have fewer diseases than members of the general population. In addition, people who are comfortable living with other people or associating with others do better than people who live alone and don't have a lot of friends. There was a study that followed single men for a year after treatment who had had myocardial infarctions. The researchers looked at diet and activities. They found the most important thing that improved their prognosis was having a dog.

In my own work, especially with cancer patients, I have seen patients do better if they had some basis in spirituality. I have known several people who seemed to have no spiritual basis whatsoever, who tended not to hold up well in life crises and during illnesses. They were certainly much more difficult to take care of than others.

On the other hand, I have also realized that certain people who were purported to have a very spiritual life—who for example went frequently to church, were publicly considered to be great church members and, in fact, seemed to lose all sense of strength in the face of crisis. When such individuals were confronted with a diagnosis of cancer, they just went completely to pieces. I was left to wonder what had happened to their spiritual belief when they reacted in that way.

In my own life, I haven't had terrific crises except possibly in the war, when we were under attack so much, the ship was hit and many people were killed. At that time, I think I handled it pretty well. I took great solace from knowing that my mother and my aunt and other members of my family were praying for me. I won't say I wasn't scared—I was. Everyone is scared under those circumstances. But I was able to handle it fairly well.

I don't know if this is a spiritual experience, but I learned that some of the things that I thought were really disastrous in my life—not getting career appointments, or getting a different appointment from the one I had wanted—turned out in the long run to be the very best thing that could have happened to me. We hear all the time about people wanting their prayers answered. I've come to accept the old saying that all prayers are answered—it is just that some of the answers are "No" instead of "Yes." When I didn't get things that I wanted badly at the time, it turned out to be the best thing. For instance, in my residency at the Lying-In Hospital, I should have gone directly from an internship there into the residency, but there was another fellow just ahead of me who Dr. Irving put in as the resident. He got me a job as assistant resident in gynecology at the Free Hospital for Women. Well, it was in that residency at the Free Hospital that I learned to be a good surgeon because we had many operations to do and mentors to help us. I've known people who have lost a job, and it was devastating for them. Maybe they lost the job through no fault of their own. But then they got another job that was much better for them, and in the long run it turned out very well. That happens to us more than we realize.

When things seem to go wrong, there can eventually emerge a feeling that maybe there was a purpose. Something was pushing the person toward accomplishing that purpose in the very best way possible. I don't know that I would say that a cancer, if it is fatal, for instance, is anything good. However, I've seen patients approach the tragedy in a way that changed their lives so that they died in a better way than they would have otherwise. I've seen many patients in our cancer support groups who, when they survived, had a completely changed value system. As one woman expressed it, "The blues are bluer and the reds are redder." They appreciated everything. They suddenly realized that some things you considered so terribly important aren't that important at all, and other things increased in importance. It could be a family, maybe a marriage—whatever. In the aftermath of serious illness, we often see that people who survive are completely changed. When they come face-to-face with the possibility that they are going to die, they see their life with a new perspective.

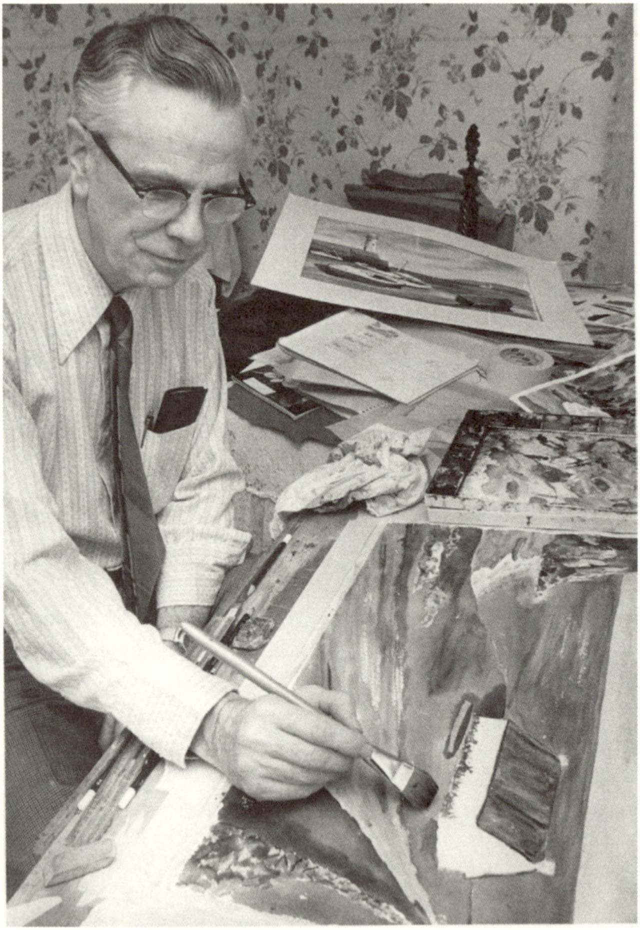

Amateur artist relaxing

7

PHOTOGRAPHY AND PAINTING

> I think watercolor painting didn't change me but brought out a hidden side of me. I always ended up doing some kind of happy paintings. We had a place at Hilton Head Island when I was busiest with my practice. We'd go down there for a week or two. I'd be very tired and tense. I remember very well one of the times that we stayed two weeks, I painted a different painting every day. At the end of the vacation, I lined them all up against the wall to see what I had done. I was completely amazed at what was so obvious. The first days' paintings were dark skies and dark oceans and storms. Each successive painting became a little more peaceful—the skies got brighter, the ocean got bluer. I was amazed because I wasn't conscious of this at all during the time that I was painting.

When I was a child, I loved to go out into the fields in our little town, go along the creeks and observe the wildlife. There were pheasants around there and rabbits and muskrats. I admired the beauty in the landscapes.

When I was in college, medical school and residency, I was too busy to do anything like that. I didn't take art in college; there weren't any courses in my small school, and I was too busy taking other things I needed.

PHOTOGRAPHY

When I finally got well established in practice during the 1950s and '60s, I got interested in photography; I used to take family pictures and portraits. I was intrigued by black-and-white photography and set up a darkroom in the basement where I could experiment with negatives. I began to develop an interest in doing wildlife photography. I wasn't interested in hunting or killing anything.

My wife had come from Canada and always wanted to go up into Algonquin Park—a wildlife preserve north of Toronto—so we took the family when the children were little. We stayed in a lodge, got a guide, went out in canoes and fished some. I saw and photographed a lot of animals—beaver and deer and mink. I was fascinated to see how the beaver could make dams that were so perfect from an engineering standpoint. I made an acquaintance with a guide up there who was also interested in wildlife photography; he had even filmed for Disney. So I went back the next year, and he and I went on a ten-day canoe trip. He could get right up close to some of the animals. He was a master, and I got wonderful shots. Every couple of years I would go up there and spend time with him; I kept getting better and better cameras and finally got a movie camera. That I enjoyed as much as anything I had ever done.

I was working very hard at medicine at the time. In fact, one of the doctors said, "It's like a religious retreat for you to go to Canada."

Sometimes on the trips I would take six to seven hundred slides and throw away the ones that weren't as good when I got back. I would end up keeping two or three hundred.

Betty went with me the first time "into the wild" and seemed to enjoy it. So the next winter, when I began to plan the summer and was thinking about going up there again, I said something to her about it.

She said, "Well, I don't believe I'll go this year."

I said, "Well, you liked it so much." She was silent. So I added, "It is so wonderful up there . . . so quiet . . . and peaceful."

She said, "Yes, too quiet! I like to hear the flushing of a toilet now and then!"

PAINTING

I was in my fifties when I began to think about painting. A couple of my physician colleagues were painting, and I enjoyed looking at their work. Because I had studied photography fairly extensively, I had learned something about design. One day, my wife and I were walking down the street in Hendersonville, North Carolina, and saw that there was an art show out on the street. I started criticizing the various paintings—areas in them I thought were poor design—and she said, "Well, if you think you are so damn good, why don't you do it yourself?"

So I started painting in watercolor. I sensed even 20 years before I retired that this would afford me something to do after retirement. I found that painting was very fulfilling and I could paint the things I liked—flowers and landscapes. I never tried to paint any wild animals, except to put some deer in some landscapes. That's a whole different ballgame.

I was so very busy I didn't have a lot of time to paint but it was relaxing when I could do it. When I'm painting,

I can't think of anything else. When I'm reading a book or watching television, other things can intrude, but when I'm painting, I can't paint and think about a sick patient.

It became apparent fairly early in my painting that my medical training, or my personality, or both, were affecting my painting greatly. In watercolor painting, one tries to be quite free with his emotions and not be precise—don't paint every brick, for example. My first instructor was an excellent watercolorist. He had won some prizes in New York, but he was getting a little old and crotchety when I started with him. One day, when I was being too careful with each stroke to suit him, he said, "Goddammit, would you stop painting as if you were operating!" After that, I tried my best to loosen up my painting and not be as precise as I would be in the operating room. When I've been able to accomplish it, the paintings have been much better. In fact, every instructor I've had has pushed me toward being looser, as the term is in art, and not being so realistic. I'm not sure it was profession so much as personality that was affecting my style—but it was associated with my being a surgeon. I remember one time that a professional artist was viewing some of my work. I had a snow scene with the path in the snow going up to the barn door from a gravel road. The pro said, "I can tell this painting was done either by a doctor or an engineer."

I said, "How can you tell?"

"Look at that path. It's just as straight as a die. You wouldn't find a path like that leading up to an old barn. It would be wiggly and banks of snow would be piled up."

Apparently, this precision has been a characteristic of my paintings through the years.

The best teacher I ever had was very abstract in her paintings. A landscape to her was a group of abstracts put together to make a landscape. But she never tried to change me into that style at all. She just showed me ways I could improve. I worked quite hard at it, because if I was going to do anything, I wanted to do it well.

I would sometimes go a lot longer without painting than I wanted to because of my medical time commitments. But I would try to take an hour or two at a time—sometimes in the evenings or on a Saturday afternoon. I didn't play golf as many doctors do. I picked watercolors because it didn't take any time to set up and, when I would stop, there was no problem cleaning brushes. In addition, if I got to the end of one painting and it was no good, I could simply tear it up and throw it away.

I think watercolor painting didn't change me but brought out a hidden side of me. I always ended up doing some kind of happy paintings. We had a place at Hilton Head Island when I was busiest with my practice. We'd go down there for a week or two. I'd be very tired and tense. I remember very well one of the times that we stayed two weeks, I painted every day a different painting. At the end of the vacation, I lined them all up against the wall to see what I had done. I was completely amazed at what was so obvious. The first days' paintings were dark skies and dark oceans and storms. Each painting became a little more peaceful—the skies got brighter, the ocean got bluer. I was amazed because I wasn't conscious of this at all during the time that I was painting.

Art, in my opinion, should generate not a sense of conflict but of peace. With so much of art now, too often one is left not feeling better, but sometimes, worse. For me, one of the greatest compliments I ever received was when I had a reception at the opening of a showing of my paintings at Mars Hill College. Quite a few of the faculty and people from around Mars Hill—I had many patients from Mars Hill—and some people from Asheville were there. During the reception, a woman who was one of the retired professors came up to me and said, "Looking at these paintings, I can see that you are a man at peace with himself." That is what I would like to be: a man at peace with himself.

Painting became a kind of therapy for me. I found it to be relaxing. In addition, I think it had something to do with creating something. When I did surgery, especially cancer surgery, I was breaking things down. Taking off a breast is a destructive thing. Creating a painting is an antidote to taking something apart and mutilating it. I noticed that among my doctor acquaintances were many avid gardeners, growing either flowers or vegetables. I used to think about that and speculate that it was partly because they wanted to create something instead of mutilate it. I really think that has a big effect on doctors.

The experience of painting solidified for me the awareness that I like beauty. I like happy situations, beaches, spring flowers. I never got into portraits, an entirely different type of art. Most people who are any good at portraits have to take quite a bit of training in that particular genre. I think I might have liked to have done it if I had had the time and the training. I did take some classes in portrait drawing and did reasonably well with them, but I never got into the actual painting.

People who study art therapy can tell from the kind of colors one used about how the artist is feeling, but I never went into the craft from an intellectual perspective. I don't know what to look for. I just know what I like. The further I went in the craft, the more I realized that certain types of art really appealed to me and said something to me.

Usually, I sketch a subject or scene first. I found it necessary to do so in order to get the design right. Many people do that to establish the picture in their mind, see where the trees fit and plan how to lead into the painting. I was always fascinated by clouds, and I was told by the instructors that I did very good skies. Many times, when the sky was an important part of the painting, I would design the whole painting so that the viewer's eye traveled completely around the painting with the help of the sky. The sky is not just something that appears with two clouds, but the arrangement of the clouds and the brights and darks in the sky have a big effect on the painting. The Dutch painters were masters of skies. Because Holland is so flat, there is a great deal of sky in almost all of their paintings.

I learned the importance of this from my teachers and then learned further from experience. Sometimes I might make a cloud that looked fine until somebody pointed out that there was a face in it, or that there was a nose sticking out, or that it looked like a dog or something else. Then that aberration would become the only thing I could see in the painting.

Many times, the images came out of my head. Somebody would look at one of my landscapes or pictures of a lake and would say, where is this? I would point to my head and say, "Up here."

I might see different things and, in my mind, put them together. This piece of river would go well with that mountain I saw when I was on vacation.

Much of my painting material came from recalling things that I'd seen that gave me ideas. Wouldn't it be nice if nature looked like that? To me, it is all about imagery. Maybe that is why at Life After Cancer I've been effective at leading imagery instruction.

If I was doing one-on-one teaching, sometimes I would go out to the home of a patient who was too sick to come in, and I would do an imagery session. I would ask, "What's a favorite place?" If it was the mountains, I could describe a mountain glade. I could describe the seashore because I've painted it a lot—the sea oats waving the colors. I could call up through my own mind the image and then describe it to the cancer patient. This would ideally project the patient into that visual setting. This taught the patients that they controlled the power of visualization. They would then be taught to visualize T cells ingesting cancer cells and the cancer getting smaller and smaller. A great deal of original research was done in this area. The studies demonstrated that it was important to see the cancer being torn up and destroyed. The investigators told of a case of a woman who didn't get anywhere with the imagery. She was envisioning raindrops coming down and splattering on the tumor. They got her to envision a bear coming in and tearing up the cells, and she began to get results. We had a patient very successful with the technique. When she was a little girl her father had a machete hanging on the wall. He was proud of it. She was terrified of it. After she learned the imagery role, she saw herself going to the wall and passionately swinging the machete, tearing up the cells.

VISION LOSS

When I was in my mid to late seventies, the eyesight in one eye went out because of an optic nerve disease. There was no treatment available for it. I was watching a basketball game on TV and noticed that there was an area where I couldn't see well, and I thought my glasses were dirty. I went in to wash my glasses and came back. I still couldn't see in that area, and then I started squinting with one eye and then the other and found the problem was in my left eye. Medical consultants assured me that the eyesight was okay in the other eye and was expected to stay unaffected. I could still drive and do most of my usual activities. I had already retired, so I was not doing surgery.

A few years later on Thanksgiving morning, I woke up and looked around the room and said, "Oh, I know what this is." A retinologist saw me in the emergency room that very morning and said, "Yes, it's in the other eye."

At that time, my vision was 20/400; 20/200 is legally blind. I had enough peripheral vision so I could get around without having any trouble, but I could no longer drive or read. The ophthalmologist said that at Duke they had devised an operation for this. It was in the very experimental stages. I went down and had a full day's testing. They were very honest about it. They said they hadn't done many procedures using this new technique. If they operated on me, I would be the ninth one. Nobody had gotten any worse after it, and some seemed to improve a good bit. They would do surgery on my eyes if I understood all of this and wanted it done. I said I thought I did because, if there was any chance of improving, it would be good, and if something went wrong, I was at an age where I wouldn't have to live with it very long. It was better to experiment on somebody my age than on somebody who is forty.

So, I had the operation the next day. Gradually, my eyesight came back to 20/200, which was very good, in comparison to my preoperative vision. It has now gotten somewhat worse again. Interestingly enough, after doing 25 or 30 such surgeries, the Duke team decided that it didn't do much good. Close up, I can see fairly well, like the computer screen or the TV screen. I can watch football, basketball and baseball. I don't see football plays very well; I lose the ball, but I've gotten pretty smart at watching different passes thrown. If I watch the receiver, even though I can't see him catch the ball, I can see that he got it from his actions.

One of the things that bothers me the most is I have great trouble seeing faces at any distance at all. People speak from 10 or 15 feet away in a crowd, at a party, or at the theatre, and I don't have any idea who they are. If it is a person I see a lot, I get to know their body English very well. Some people who know I have this vision problem will tell me who they are, but it can be embarrassing at times.

When my eyesight worsened, it became difficult to paint. After I got over the operation, I tried to do some watercolors. I found I couldn't mix the paints to get the color I wanted, and I couldn't really paint well at arm's length. I got a few things started, but they weren't going well and I got pretty discouraged. In fact, that was the first time I cried in many years. So I just quit painting. Then I went to a meeting of the American Physicians' Art Association of which I had been president. We had yearly exhibitions with physician-artists coming from all over the country. That year, there was a painting in the exhibit that had been done on the computer. The fellow who did it wasn't there, but I got his name, called him up and talked to him, and decided that I would like to try it because, at that time, I knew I could see if I was close to the television screen.

I didn't want to buy a lot of expensive equipment. It was a lot more expensive than it is now. I looked all over the area for anyone else doing computer art and finally found a man at the community college down in Marion, North Carolina. He was head of the art department there. They were teaching this because there was a great demand for computer graphics. He was kind enough to arrange to spend an hour or two with me in the computer room after classes. He showed me how to do it. When I finally decided I would be able to manage the technique on my own, I was ready to buy my equipment. Whenever I got stuck, I'd call him and he would talk over the phone, or come up to Asheville and work with me for a couple of hours.

Computer art is satisfying when the product is finished and it is good. It's more tedious doing it because it is more difficult by far to control the cursor than it is to paint with a brush. However, certain things are a lot easier with a computer than with a brush. For instance, if I made a stroke I didn't like, or decided the color wasn't right, I could simply hit a button, and the stroke would disappear. That is not possible in watercolor. If I decide a tree is in the wrong place, I can move it over somewhere else where I want it. It is easier to correct mistakes by far. On the other hand, I find drawing the outline of a boat quite difficult. I took a photograph of subject material that I liked very much, scanned it on to the computer and then changed it as I would want it to be. With my eyesight failing, painting on the computer was easier than starting from scratch.

A painting I did of Peggy's Cove, Newfoundland, is a typical example of the process I follow. I'd always wanted to go there and finally did. It is in a small fishing village on the coast of Canada north of Halifax. I'd seen innumerable paintings—every artist who can get up there goes to paint. The rocks are beautiful. I took a number of photos and then picked out one with some boats and a building that I liked. I scanned it and rearranged the position of the buildings and boats. I made a channel out to the sea in the rocks, which had been solid all the way across, and moved a lighthouse over from another picture onto the tip of the rocks. After painting out several white houses that had been on those rocks and did not seem to fit, I moved and changed the color of the remaining building. The entire picture was transformed. It would have been very difficult for me, with my eyesight the way it is, to have drawn those boats exactly as they are, but I did repaint them.

Loss of some of my vision forced a looser style of painting. I painted trees differently—I painted them looser to make the feel of the branches coming in and out. To get depth, I needed to do that. I could get depth with color, too.

Although I miss being able to create watercolor paintings, learning to produce computer images has been a new challenge and has enabled me to continue to express myself in art.

8

LEAVING MEDICAL PRACTICE

The leaving of medicine did not affect my sense of identity as much as other people and I thought it would. Many times I've been asked, "Don't you miss it?" But in fact, there was that feeling of relief from the responsibility. Just recently, I was talking with one of the pediatricians in town who is also retired. He said, "You know, people are always asking me, 'What do I do to keep busy?' I tell them, 'Why do I want to keep busy?'" I never thought of it that way, but maybe that is part of what I am talking about.

TRANSITION OUT OF OBSTETRICS

For many years, I enjoyed both Ob and Gyn. I enjoyed the Ob because I was taking care of younger people—most of whom were quite happy and would have a good outcome of a pregnancy for which they would be happy. There was enough challenge with the various complications of pregnancy that I enjoyed it very much. I enjoyed practicing gynecology because of doing so much surgery. I had a feeling of accomplishment when a difficult operation went well.

As the years went by, it got a little bit more difficult to get up in the middle of the night. By then we had started a group practice, the younger doctors could take over the obstetrics and I just felt like it was time for me to ease off. I felt that my life would be better. I would have more time to do the things that I wanted. So I started saying that I would not take any new Ob patients. I would deliver some of the subsequent babies for those for whom I had previously delivered babies, but I wouldn't take on any new patients. That cut down my numbers over a period of time.

I was amazed, after I had not done any Ob for several months, suddenly to realize how many of the phone calls to my home previously had been to do with obstetrics. The number of phone calls dropped off dramatically. Sometimes, I would wake up in the morning, and, not having had a call during the night, I would pick the phone up off the hook and listen to see if there was anything wrong with it. There had been so many obstetrical questions—not only from patients, but their mothers—wanting to know if it was okay for their daughters to drive to Hendersonville or get their hair done or something like that. There is very little of those types of questions in gynecology, so it was an easier life physically by far. I didn't have to do the prenatal work or spend so much time in the hospital with patients in labor. I saw so many more Gyn patients that my gross charges increased rather than decreased. I enjoyed doing more gynecology. At the same time, I was getting more and more involved with cancer patients.

After leaving obstetrics, besides having more time with my family, I did some community service. Of course,

I also had a lot of time when I just wanted to sleep. I can think of many times when I would go to bed at 7:30 at night because I had been up three or four nights in a row and I didn't know if I was going to have to get up that night. If I went to bed at 7:30 and I got up at midnight to deliver a baby, I would have had some sleep. So, pretty much, my practice had ruled what I did.

NEW DOCTORS

The first thing I noticed about the younger physicians coming in was that they depended a lot more on laboratory work than I did. In fact, I used to caution them that if the laboratory work did not agree with what they thought, to be very careful because they might well be right, and the laboratory work could be misleading. Not only did I see more dependence on laboratory work than I thought necessary, but also more laboratory work being done than I thought was necessary. However, I tried to remember that they were just out of training, and that probably was the reason for it. There was more laboratory work to be done and more known about its interpretation than in my day. It used to concern me some that maybe I was just plain behind the times for not thinking that all that laboratory work was necessary.

I found it good to have the younger doctors around because, not infrequently, I would go and ask them, "What did they say in your training about doing such and such? Do you think this is better than that?" It was really a help to me to have them there.

New physicians brought a variety of personalities on the scene. Some of them were very interested in the business end of medicine, and some weren't interested in it at all. Some were interested in the emotional side of their patients, and some were not interested at all.

As I look back on my internship—at both the surgeons under whom I was working and the people who were teaching me—they covered the same set of personality characteristics that physicians seem to have now. Some of them were interested more in money than anything else. Some of them couldn't care less about the money and were interested in the patients, and some were interested in the scientific part of the disease. I don't think that has changed any.

They had some new techniques that I worked hard to pick up. Laparoscopy, for instance, came in relatively late in my career, but I went and took courses so that I could do it. Laser didn't come in until I was about ready to retire, so I never did any of that.

But I made a point of learning colposcopy for positive Pap smears. Even though I was close to retirement, I took courses to get proficient in that.

Colposcopy is a method of looking at the cervix through a series of lenses. If a Class III PAP smear detected dysplasia, it was possible to pick out the exact part of the cervix that was involved and biopsy it. Sometimes it might be possible even to eliminate it with a biopsy if it was small and early enough. When I retired, I was approached by individuals at the Health Department to do a clinic for women found to have abnormal Pap smears. I told them I would be very glad to do so, but I wanted them to pay my malpractice insurance premiums because they were much too high to pay by myself without any income coming in from it. They didn't think they could do that, so that never came to fruition.

TRANSITION OUT OF GYNECOLOGY

For a long time, I had a rule with myself that I would not try to practice after I shouldn't be practicing—I wanted to practice good medicine until the last day. I wouldn't operate longer than I should, in terms of age—which does happen. I remember when I was a "young" 50-year-old, I would sometimes walk by operating rooms with other physicians and would pass a room with a seventy-year-old surgeon performing a procedure. I remember hearing comments like, "Why doesn't that old guy know when to quit?" I made a mental note that I didn't want to be guilty of provoking such disapprobation, and I especially didn't want to jeopardize my patients.

I think I was about 68 years old when I decided that the thing that bothered me about the surgery in the latter years was the post-operative care, which had become very scientific. Noting the laboratory work that some physicians were using—even though I often didn't see the point or think it was absolutely necessary—I began to wonder if I wasn't the one who was out of step. Also, when I was 68, I was getting fatigued after some operations, and my dexterity was not what it had been. So I stopped operating. I kept on assisting other surgeons. I was quite in demand as an assistant, and I enjoyed being in the operating room, but I was somewhat relieved to get out from under the feeling of responsibility.

I still had a big gynecology office practice, which mostly consisted of older patients coming back for checks or coming in when something went wrong. By older, I mean patients I had seen over a period of time. Many of them had become like old friends. I enjoyed seeing all of them and asking about the kids I had delivered. That kept me in the swing, so to speak, and kept me with people I enjoyed. There again, it was nice to have, as time went on, the younger fellows there, because I could step out and ask them if there was anything new that they knew of in this particular situation or that, because I couldn't keep up.

As time went on, and I was just doing office work and some surgical assisting, my practice got smaller because obviously there were very few young women coming to see me when they knew they couldn't continue for long as my patients. It got so that it wasn't remunerative at all. I kept up with expenses, but somehow it just grew on me that this was getting to be the time to retire. I can't really explain what happened—it just seemed right to stop. Even after I closed the office and stopped practicing, I was asked on several occasions to come back and assist different people, especially if they were providing care to old patients of mine. Hospitals put in a rule that I couldn't assist unless I had malpractice insurance, so that ended that part of it. Of course, I kept up my counseling work with Life After Cancer. I was still very active in that and could do more in that line.

TRANSITIONS OBSERVED IN SEXUALITY

What I saw as I looked back on my obstetrics-gynecologic practice over the years was a complete change, step-by-step, in sexual mores—attitudes about sexuality.

In the beginning, when I was in the Navy in Atlanta, there was a large problem of dysmenorrhea and women complained of "frigidity." I came to realize that at least part of it was due to the fact that mothers were so afraid their daughters would get pregnant—such a disaster if they did—that they made sexuality appear as unpleasant as possible. I believed this accounted for a lot of the frigidity. I did not neglect the role the male partner might be playing in the problem.

Dysmenorrhea

I saw young women, age 14-15 to late 20s, missing work and school because of dysmenorrhea—painful menstrual periods. Some of the same young women, three to four months after marriage, complained of frigidity.

A lot of times, the girls with severe dysmenorrhea would stay home from school several days a month. Their mothers were the ones who would say that intercourse was the "worst thing in the world." The same mothers would instill fear of pregnancy and anything connected with it.

Menses were seen as the "curse" from parents—fathers included—and with it came fear of pregnancy. In the last years of my practice, dysmenorrhea had almost disappeared—perhaps due to modern analgesics to some degree, but also to a change in female self-perception.

I recall a 15-year-old who came in with a big hefty mother like a linebacker. The daughter was just a little cringy thing. The girl was missing school four to five days a month. The mother answered all my questions that I asked her daughter. My nurse and I took the patient into the examination room without the mother present and found that everything was fine.

In the consultation room afterwards, trying to reassure her that menses are normal, I said, "Actually, if you have pain with a period, it means you ovulate, and if you don't have pain, you may not be ovulating. So, you see, this is a good sign that when you are older, it will be medically okay to get pregnant and have children."

"Yes! And then she'll vomit the whole nine months, just like I did!" her mother interjected.

Yes, I said to myself, *she sure will.*

Frigidity

When I first started practicing, seeing women in Atlanta in the Navy, at a postoperative examination they would say, "Am I okay down there?"

"Yeah, sure," I would say, until I understood the deeper purpose behind the question.

"But I never reach a climax."

One patient was a very intelligent woman who had a husband with a good job. She reported that, after her first baby, she began wearing flannel nightgowns and would keep the baby up till late so everyone would be tired. "So he'll stay away from me," she said. "But part of me doesn't like it." I sent her to a colleague who was an excellent psychiatrist. Early in my practice I began sending a lot of cases to him. Our offices were in the same wing of the building, and we shared a common hall. One day I was in the shared hallway. His doorway opened and she stuck her head out. "I want to tell you," she said, "I burned the flannel nighties, and the baby goes to bed at five o'clock!"

I got a letter from the psychiatrist about another patient—a report about a woman I had referred. He said, "Easiest case you ever sent me! All I had to do was tell her husband to take a shower!"

His style was finding out about the source of the problems. He said that so much was due to the fact that the women, as girls, had been told "all this"—so many negative things about their sexuality—to "protect" them from pregnancy. One of the things some fathers started doing later on was not to allow the girls to go on a date alone with a boy. "He must think I'm a latent whore," the fifteen-year-old girl would muse.

Change in sexual practices

As years went on, there were fewer patient complaints about dysmenorrhea and frigidity among the younger women. Things had "loosened up" to the point that they were asking, not complaining, about their husbands wanting them to have oral intercourse . . . was that healthy? Change in social mores affected the attitudes of young women toward their bodies. "Am I okay down there?" shifted to "Why am I not reaching a climax with intercourse?" These changes seemed to come in 15-year intervals.

Then, after ten or fifteen years, the focus of questions changed. Patients started addressing new issues. "My husband is interested in my performing oral sex for him. Is that all right?" became the new question, shifting to the 15-20-year-olds. Again, I said it was okay if that is what she also wanted. The practices became more and more liberal. The pendulum would swing back and forth, but not very far back. I said, "It may be a step to 'normal' intercourse. Consensus is the important thing—whatever both partners want."

Birth control pills and other contraception brought freedom from dysmenorrhea and frigidity but liberalized promiscuity.

In those days we had to do a Wasserman—test for syphilis—before marriage. The couple would come in to be tested premaritally, and I would always do an examination. I never had a patient in the office whom I didn't examine. For a long time, most were virgins, and then it became fewer and fewer. It got to be that I stopped teaching about intercourse. They knew more than I did!

Then, after another fifteen-year interval, it seemed that promiscuity had become common. Now young folks openly travel together, spend weekends together, take up residence together and of course start families with unmarried partners.

RETIREMENT

The leaving of medicine did not affect my sense of identity as much as other people and I thought it would. Many times

I've been asked, "Don't you miss it?" But in fact, there was that feeling of relief from the responsibility. Just recently, I was talking with one of the pediatricians in town who is also retired. He said, "You know, people are always asking me, 'What do I do to keep busy?' I tell them, 'Why do I want to keep busy?'" I never thought of it that way, but maybe that is part of what I am talking about.

The transition was easier than I thought it would be. I missed the operating room, and, for a while, I missed the people whom I had seen so much, but I didn't really suffer in the way some people do who quit business and just seem to be lost. I was doing a lot of painting—I enjoyed that. Betty and I traveled. We started going to places we hadn't been before, like South Africa, Australia and Greece.

I retired the first of July, 1985—three months before I turned 72. As I think back over the fifty years that I was associated with medicine, either in medical school, or in residency, or in the practice of medicine, I have a feeling of great thankfulness that I was so privileged. I was happy as I aged to turn medicine over to someone else.

Since I've retired, I have known many retired men, and it's interesting to see how various people handle their retirement. It's my observation that people tend to pretty much go on with the same types of lives they had in their business or profession. People who were interested in community activities and charitable institutions while they were active in business or professions tend to continue to be involved in those areas. They are in great demand after they retire and, in fact, are sought after by various charitable institutions to work with them. Others, who were interested in reading, read a great deal more. Those who were interested in physical activities, such as golf, play a lot more golf. Many couples start to travel. Betty and I would take fairly long trips and found this very interesting, but in the last few years found them too tiring at any length.

Some of the people whom I knew and who retired went into a depression because they no longer felt needed. Maybe they had been in a very responsible job, were looked up to by many people and suddenly did not feel important. I felt that these people did not attempt to do things to bring new purpose to their lives. There is plenty of activity to do. There is plenty of charity work waiting, and if that is not interesting, there are retirement classes at the colleges. Many people are very happy to take all the classes that they can. And the Elderhostels! Although I've lectured for them on the emotional part of cancer, I've never gone in for them in my own retirement, but some people find them extremely rewarding.

It has been interesting to see the occasional situation where the man relishes the retirement and the wife does not. I think of one couple who moved down here from Chicago where the man had been a very successful person and very busy. He was just enjoying retirement to the fullest—playing golf and playing cards at the country club. The wife was very upset by retirement and went into quite a decline. In Chicago, she had been, you might say, a granddame and chairwoman of this art committee and that symphony committee and all sorts of charities and charity balls. Down here, she missed having all that to do and really became quite depressed. That is not what one would ordinarily think is the situation in retirement. I think that everyone should start to contemplate retirement long before the exact time. Too many people make no advance plans.

For myself, I had my photography interest, then my painting interest, and I kept my interests in the emotional side of cancer. Because of my work at Life After Cancer, I studied research papers, kept up with the advances in cancer and continued to work in the field. I used to go to medical meetings to pick up the latest in cancer treatments, especially the latest in research on the mind-body connection. This had a positive, stimulating effect for me. For awhile, I continued going to some of the medical meetings that I had attended regularly over the years because I still saw friends of mine who would come from various places to these meetings. Now there is almost no one left in my age group who is going to these meetings.

Financial planning is certainly in order if one is going to enjoy retirement. In the late '60s, the government allowed medical practices to incorporate and thereby set up pension and profit-sharing plans. What money I was able to accumulate was after taxes rather than before. Nowadays, doctors are retiring with retirement money that has accumulated tax-free, albeit taxable at the time of use. This makes a great deal of difference. The period of time when I was able to put money into a pension/profit-sharing plan was after the time when my income was at its highest. Even so, it amounted to a fair amount when compared to my earlier efforts to save for retirement.

The people who have no interest outside of whatever they are doing—medicine, law or other fields—do suffer considerably from a forced retirement. One of the things I have seen in the past—not so much now—is doctors practicing after they were not really able to do good medicine. They didn't want to retire because they didn't have any other interests.

The question of what the older retired generation can contribute to society is an open question as far as I am concerned. Certainly experience counts, and there are some areas where someone with a vast amount of experience can be very helpful. The problem is that if one gets set in one's ideas, it is very difficult to keep up with and use the knowledge and ideas well because of the way that things are moving so rapidly.

I am amazed, for instance, at the knowledge that my older grandchildren have on certain subjects. I shudder to think of the problems that they are going to have to face in government and in living in the future. Some of the troubles seem to be almost insoluble—certainly world issues and the challenges of the environment. The advice I might have on that would not, I think, be very applicable.

I do think that one of the problems the world faces in the generation coming up is greed. One way or another, greed seems to affect so many people and therefore their countries. It keeps people and countries from doing what is best for the whole because "somebody's ox is gored" every time you try to improve something.

I see people that have retired with millions and millions of dollars, and they want it right there. They won't give it away. The government is going to take it away from them when they die, but they don't figure that. That is one type of greed. Then there's the—let me phrase it like this—climbing up somebody's back to get on top. In other words, as we used to say in the Navy, "Pull up the gangplank, I'm aboard." I don't know exactly what words to use to express how I feel. All you have to do is look at the foolishness of college athletics. Colleges are doing everything they can to get an athlete there. A professor is working his tail off trying to teach something, but they pay a coach a million dollars a year.

I've known a couple of guys who got out of Harvard Law School and got into the big, big law firms in New York—the very prestigious ones. They worked for years as slaves, literally, until ten or eleven o'clock at night, and were paid essentially nothing. And finally, if they didn't make anybody mad and did all the work, they finally got to be one of the partners and begin to make some money.

But they were poverty-stricken, literally, for years. In the meantime, the guys at the top were making millions. Perhaps the generation coming up will find ways for more fairness.

One thing which has come to the fore since my own retirement at age 72 is the fact that doctors are retiring earlier and earlier. When I first entered the field of medicine, many doctors worked until they died, especially family practitioners in small towns. In my early days of practice in the 1950s, we saw people working much longer than they should have. They weren't mentally and emotionally capable anymore, but they just wouldn't stop. Of course, in those days there were no tax-free retirement accounts such as 401K, and they were not allowed to have pension and profit sharing plans like industry did. This was one of the reasons that the doctors fought going under Social Security. Statistics showed that doctors lived only a few years after they retired, and it was felt by the medical community that if they were under Social Security, they would put a lot more money into it than they ever got out of it. But now all that is changed. With the pension and profit-sharing plans of the medical corporations, doctors are able to accumulate money to retire on and they are retiring earlier and earlier.

I know one doctor who retired at age fifty. Many of my younger colleagues are retiring at 60 and 62. There are several reasons for the "early" retirement. One is that they are all having problems with the rules that are being set for them. The insurance companies really interfere with their practice, and so does the government through Medicare and Medicaid. This interference is particularly frustrating for a person who has practiced for years, doing what he or she thought best, without interference from outside lay people. Now with HMOs, there is a great deal of pressure on physicians to practice the way the executives of the HMOs think they should.

Another factor in early retirement is that it is very difficult to slow down because overhead expenses are so high. The doctor has to work hard and, in some instances, feels that he is just working to pay the overhead. The record-keeping alone, which insurance requires, necessitates at least one person who does nothing but insurance in most offices. In any group practice, with any number of doctors at all, it is imperative to have an office manager who can keep up with the various rules and filing requirements. These are in addition to the nurses and secretaries and physician extenders. When a physician tries to cut down, the overhead does not decrease proportionately—it eats him up, making him consider stopping instead.

9

REFLECTIONS

> I was brought up in a family that had a pretty sound value system. As long as I can remember, I understood that honesty was the thing to do and that serving others was a laudable practice. I don't think I ever put money high up on the list. I did want enough money to feel secure in retirement. I saw my parents struggle through the Depression and end up with barely enough money to live comfortably in their retirement. That made me determined not to earn a lot of money and then just waste it.

As I look at medicine today and think back over the 60 years or so that I have been associated with it, I naturally see some things that I feel should be changed. At the same time, there are many things that have shown tremendous improvement. Medicine today is extremely complex. There is so much research going on. The field of genetics has had so many advances. Various diseases are treated differently from the way they were treated just a short time ago. New diseases are cropping up all the time. Almost monthly—or certainly yearly—there is a vast amount of knowledge that the doctor has to assimilate and use in the day-to-day seeing of patients.

I suppose that the many very fine changes in medicine—such as the ability to thread catheters up the veins and into the heart with various electronic devices carried with them to see exactly what is going on—have saved many lives.

However, the advances have come with some price. Medicine is very expensive for the patient and for the doctors too. Frequently the equipment is very expensive but becomes obsolete rapidly, so that it has to be continually replaced to stay at the top of the field. The doctors are so specialized now that they seldom see the same patient over a period of time, and the patient in some ways suffers from this in that there is less of a personal aspect to medicine. In many ways, it is now more a business than a profession.

PRIMARY CARE

One of the things that stands out is the predominance and fast-growing importance of the primary care physician. I've always had great admiration for the good family doctors in light of what they have to know and can do. A great amount of responsibility is placed on the practice of primary medicine by insurance companies who do not want any more people going to specialists than they can help. There is more training in the medical schools to orient future physicians to primary care. I know that at Harvard, students spend a great deal of time in clinics in the city of Boston under the tutelage of carefully-selected primary care physicians.

The time is coming—and I would like to see it—when the postgraduate residencies in primary care will be extended. Now, most of them last for three years, and I think that, with the vast amount of knowledge that these young people have to absorb, they need more than three years of training. For instance, a surgeon usually takes five years to get surgical credentials. If he or she goes on from there into a subspecialty of cardiovascular surgery or oncology surgery, two or three more years are added to those five. Certainly, if the surgical subspecialist needs five to eight years of training, the family practitioner, in my opinion, with all the things that must be learned, needs up to five years training to be adequate for the job. The primary care physician has more responsibility now and will have more in the future, positioned by the health maintenance organizations (HMOs) as the gatekeeper who decides whether or not a patient needs to go to a specialist. Furthermore, additional experience and training is needed in the interpretation of laboratory work and X-rays and other imaging.

The challenge for family practitioners is deciding what they can handle and what they can't. Longer training, it seems to me, would help this. In my practice, I occasionally had patients referred from a general practitioner, whom I thought surely knew how to handle the problem in his own office, and then I would not get a patient referred who really should have been referred, for example, with a cancer that was growing undetected.

I think in the matter of physician education, medical schools have to increase what they are doing now. Many of the schools, to their credit, are bringing some of the alternative types of medicine into the curriculum. I feel it is extremely important for the medical student to be well grounded in nutrition, acupuncture, chiropractic and other types of alternative medicine—and certainly psychosomatic medicine, the study of how the mind can affect the body. These basics have been neglected for too long. I never had anything on nutrition in medical school or in my training. Of course, we were taught what vitamins were and what a vitamin deficiency would be, but nothing about the deleterious effect of a bad diet and high cholesterol intake. It doesn't mean that the physician will have to be able to do acupuncture, but there seems to be no question now that there are certain cases in which acupuncture is an advantage. The modern physician should know the benefits and send the patient to someone skilled in providing the technique.

SPECIALTIES AND SUBSPECIALTIES

In the past few years, group practice of varying kinds has proliferated extremely rapidly. There are multispecialty groups with doctors in a variety of disciplines working together, for example, internists, Ob-Gyns, pediatricians and surgeons. More common are single-specialty groups. The push for larger groups started for several reasons. One is that doctors got tired of being on call constantly and wanted time off. With three or four obstetricians operating together, one member of the group could be in the hospital at certain times, while others are in the office.

Recently, it has become imperative to be in a group because of the terrific overhead costs of a practice. A physician can't practice now without having a person who does nothing but the insurance forms. To sort out rules of Medicare and Medicaid, the forms for private insurance and the policies of HMOs, a full-time employee is needed who knows all the ins and outs of this. Besides secretaries and nurses, there must be a business manager to keep up with the running of the office in a setting of changing tax situations and changing government regulations. With a group practice, the same amount of overhead can take care of several doctors instead of one. Furthermore, multiple physicians can share costly equipment in a group practice rather than each needing to buy a separate item.

One of the problems with large medical groups is that the patients sometimes lose any sort of a personal touch. They see one person one time and a different person at another. This could lead to problems in treatment, if one doctor doesn't know what the other has done. Even though there are records available, there have been some mistakes made on this basis.

There is another form of medical care coming to the fore now, and that is specialty groups who work together in the care of a patient. The cancer patient might have a radiologist, a radiation oncologist, a medical oncologist, a surgeon, possibly an interested family practitioner or internist, and possibly a psychologist or psychosomatic specialist. They manage the case together. The team meets and reviews the whole situation, decides on the appropriate treatments, and then keeps reviewing the situation of the patient as a group. Where this team approach is being done, it is working very, very well, and the statistics are showing that it is very valuable. I hope that this will be studied and will lead to more and more medical problems handled in this manner. For instance, I can see great value in a cardiovascular group meeting and discussing particular patients from all sides.

Time is one problem. People are busy. It is hard to get them together. For it to work, the clinicians must want to do it. Personalities can be very difficult in medicine. There are different attitudes about specialization; if individual egos keep getting in the way—somebody doesn't want to have somebody else interfering with his case—it won't work. In addition, there are financial questions to work out—who is getting paid for what?

The benefit to the patient is having more than one person's ideas on the case. Somebody might know something that somebody else doesn't. Another might bring up something that has been missed. It is good for a physician to be exposed to individuals with different training in medicine—to learn that everything doesn't go just the way you've been taught to do it. There are advantages in having different ideas come into the equation.

I thought subspecialities were a good development in medicine because the more the subspecialist knew about something, the better the care could be. They could know more, read more, go to more meetings and keep up better than I could in their specified area. I was trying to keep up with everything. There are two sides to all specialty issues, however.

A woman came to me with pain in her coccyx area. She had seen an orthopedic surgeon, who sent her to a proctologist, who sent her to me. When I found her cancer in the uterus, she said, "Why, if that area takes up so little space, couldn't some of the other doctors at least have done a pelvic examination?"

A mother of a friend of mine got sick at age 75. She had an internist whom she asked a lot of questions, "What was the matter?" She was in a lot of abdominal pain. She was finally brought to Asheville to see the best gastroenterologist. He and his associates thought it might be pancreatitis. Finally she got an ultrasound. The ultrasound showed cancer of the ovaries. I was called to the hospital to see her. No one of the specialists had ever done a pelvic examination. The tumor was easy to feel.

Sometimes physicians can be too subspecialized. They should be doctors first and specialists second.

PHYSICIAN LIABILITY

Before I retired in 1985, I saw a drastic change in physicians' rates for malpractice coverage. It was a change in medicine, in general, and obstetrics, in particular. Nature is not perfect in what it does reproductively, and things go wrong, some of which are possibly the fault of the physician, but frequently they are not. The public now has the attitude that everything should go right, and a perfect baby should be the result. If not, someone must pay no matter whose actual fault it is or whether any person or institution is at fault at all. Some people feel they should be compensated simply for something not going right. Too many juries, unfortunately, seem to be taking the attitude that it doesn't cost anybody anything anyway because the insurance companies are paying for it. But of course it does cost people, including themselves, a lot of money because the premiums have to be paid on the insurance.

Neurosurgeons and anesthesiologists are other specialists with a high rate of lawsuits and, consequently, high rates for insurance coverage. This pushes medical costs up. The hospitals would typically be called into these suits, with the anesthesiologists, the nurses and everyone else participating in the patient's care included as parties in the negligence. Large settlements made by the hospital cannot be known by a jury hearing the trial of the physician, so the payments are compounded. The whole thing is completely out of hand.

Orthopedics is another specialty with high malpractice rates. When an individual gets a very bad break in a limb, the nature of the break sometimes means that there is not 100% use of the extremity again. Regardless of where the patient lives in the country, if he can show that he can't function thus-and-so, then the physician gets sued.

I don't know if general surgeons get sued as much as the Obs and the "orthopods." A lot can happen in an abdominal operation; there can be real mistakes—but nobody knows about it because they can't see them.

The results in medicine are judged by patient expectations. I suppose this could partly be blamed on a physician not explaining the procedure carefully enough. Take a new patient in Ob who comes in happy, her first pregnancy, three months along. The physician does not want to sit down with her and tell her all the horrible things that could happen before the pregnancy is over. The rate of those things is one in one thousand, but they could happen, and if they happen to her, she would be unhappy.

There is evidence that a lot of malpractice cases are started by the attorneys. There have been studies done, one in Detroit years ago, where it was found that certain lawyers were paying certain nurses and orderlies to report to them the names of people when they thought something had gone wrong in the treatment. Then they would call the patient and say, "You know, you have the possibility of a lawsuit." There was a study in which patients were asked what started them on the road to suing, and a substantial percentage said, "We never thought of suing until someone told us we had a suit."

This is affecting the conduct of medicine. It's causing a great many laboratory tests, which are not necessary because the physician has thoughts of getting up on the witness stand and being asked by an attorney, "Why didn't you do such and such a test?"

If he were to answer, "Well, it didn't seem to be indicated at the time," the lawyer may take that fact and turn it around to appear that the doctor was not taking good care of the patient. So, the physicians load all the charts with all sorts of lab work, just in case. If an intestinal obstruction is suspected, for example, just a simple X-ray of the abdomen at a glance might tell if that diagnosis is present. Yet sometimes, if I sent a patient for that X-ray, the radiologist, for fear of missing something, would report that there was no evidence of an intestinal obstruction but would put a sentence on his report that a CT scan would be advisable. Well, with that on there—despite knowing well that isn't needed— if the record ever got in court that a full CT scan wasn't ordered, where would I be?

PREVENTATIVE MEDICINE

I've been interested in the last few years in the preventive aspect of medicine. We are taught in medical school how to treat diseases, but recently there has been a big push to try to prevent people from getting certain diseases. Early in my medical career, preventive medicine consisted of inoculations and vaccinations, and great strides were made in those to the point that some diseases, such as polio and measles and other childhood diseases, have been almost abolished. At that time, there was great pressure to improve sewage systems and water supplies, and there was a focus on testing wells. Cows were tested for various diseases transmitted in milk. Now that such past epidemics have been pretty well conquered, the emphasis has changed to healthful living.

However, there has developed a complacency about having children get inoculations for various things like polio. Around the world, some of the diseases that have almost been knocked out are beginning to make a comeback. In this country, at least inoculation is required to go to school.

We know so much more about the damage an unhealthy diet, smoking and lack of exercise do. The push now is to get people to live those healthier lives. This would cut down some of the diseases which are major causes of illness and death—like heart disease, strokes and cancer. There is plenty of knowledge. The problem is to get people to use this knowledge and live the way they should.

The National Academy of Sciences has figures to show that if there were absolutely no cigarette smoking, cancer would be cut down 33% and heart disease would be reduced by 33%.

It is true that the overall amount of cigarette smoking is less, but it is also true that young people—especially women—are smoking more. In just the last few years the incidence of lung cancer in women has passed the incidence of breast cancer.

I was at a very large cancer conference several years ago where some of the top researchers in the cancer field reported their works. I noticed that a good many of them were very despondent about the fact that they were giving their lives to work on this, and yet people were just going on and smoking and living lifestyles that promoted cancer.

A great deal of research has been applied to how to educate young people to live healthy lives. It has to be a matter of peer-to-peer talking. We can show these people all sorts of figures and talk to them, and they say, "Yes, that's interesting, but it's not going to happen to me." But if we could make it cool to eat a good diet, not smoke and get plenty of exercise, youth would pick it up. How you do that, I don't know. It would help if more of our sports stars who are so much in the limelight would get into this. The few who are lecturing on this probably have more effect than we know, but there is not enough of it going on. I would like, for instance, to see some of the athletes who are role models for younger people take this more seriously. It is not as bad as it used to be, but it bothers me tremendously to see professional ball players stand up at the plate with a big wad of chewing tobacco in their cheek. I wish they would stop showing on television the shots of players sitting in the dugout spitting all the time. I wish they would take seriously the example they are setting.

Another one of our greatest problems is drunk driving. There again, we constantly read on the sports pages of the athlete being arrested for drunk driving, and occasionally, a death resulting. If public figures would set a better example, it would be a great help in cutting down some of the things we know are so deleterious to health.

An aspect of preventive medicine that I find extremely interesting has come up in recent years—the relaxation response. It consists of teaching people the ability to relax, meditate, take some time to withdraw from the hurly-burly of life and reflect on themselves. Research has proven that people who do this have fewer diseases—especially serious diseases—than the general population. Some of the medical schools are beginning to teach this and have clinics in relaxation techniques and meditation.

Reducing stress, as a preventive health measure, has been studied for some time now. We first thought of stress as a precursor to heart trouble. We know now it may have something to do with other diseases. It is interesting to follow certain people who have had conditions—such as arthritis and heart disease and cancer—over a period of time sequentially. We find that typically they have not liked their jobs and have had a lot of stress in family life. Everybody has stress, but learning how to handle it is a helpful preventive of certain diseases.

Many technical advances are now used for the purpose of preventing disease rather than in treating it. During my early practice years, we were completely focused on treating various diseases. Now we have much information to indicate who is at high risk for certain diseases. Therefore, we can use our tools to actually prevent some diseases from ever occurring. These tools include the Pap smear to detect cancer of the cervix, radiological techniques for diagnosis, ultrasound studies and vascular advances, such as injecting dye into the blood vessels to see whether a coronary artery is getting calcium in it.

Magnetic resonance imaging (MRI) procedures and computerized axial tomography (CAT) scans have enabled us to see into the body and have greatly diminished the necessity for exploratory surgery. In many cases, it is possible to see if there is a brain tumor or a cyst in the brain and what it is like—malignant or not. The studies can be used to follow bone repair. This has enabled orthopedists to better treat certain types of fractures.

We can tell with certain tests that a woman has a 75% chance of having breast cancer because of her genetics, or, in contrast, that she does not have much chance at all of getting breast cancer. With amniocentesis, which involves taking amniotic fluid out from around the fetus, we can tell whether the fetus has genetic disorders or certain other diseases and act accordingly. With ultrasound, multiple pregnancies can be diagnosed and anomalies can be detected early—such as anencephaly (absence of the skull and most of the brain) and certain difficulties with the spinal cord. Such findings would guide intervention options and timing. These things have added to the ability to prevent disease or to head it off when it is still not serious.

Chemotherapy has done much to change the treatment of cancer and is being improved upon daily with new drugs and new attacks on the cancer cell in that way. It is very heartening to see the improvements in this. Yearly the overall cancer cure rate is slowly improving for all kinds of cancer.

It is amazing to see the brilliance of some of the men and women both in research and in the teaching aspects of medicine now. There are some very bright people who make these advances of the last few years.

Sometimes I wonder, when I think of all the things that the students have to learn now and that we never even touched on in medical school, whether I could even be accepted into medical school now.

It was very discouraging to see patients doing things, such as smoking, that I knew hurt them and would lead to serious problems. Even when they knew it too, they would often not go into a healthy regimen. The fact that so many teenagers—especially girls—are starting to smoke bothers me tremendously. Not only is the young woman risking her own health, but we know that smoking leads to a high percentage of miscarriage and premature babies. Premature babies sometimes don't do well in later life. Smoking contributes to all sorts of troubles in the babies. The English studied this. Investigators claimed that they could go into a first-grade class and tell you whose mother smoked during pregnancy. The physician can tell girls the risks, and the reply is, "Well, it won't happen to me," like they have to prove that somebody older and wiser can't control their life. In addition, smoking will increase the incidence of several types of cancer—breast, uterine, prostate, lung and bladder.

On the other hand, it is interesting to observe how informed many patients are now. We're dealing with an entirely different class of patients from the ones with whom we dealt 50 years ago because television, magazines and the Internet are full of information about new treatments and new drugs. It is interesting to me to watch the morning news shows—such as Good Morning America and The Today Show. The day that the *New England Journal of Medicine*—which is one of the most prestigious and best medical periodicals—comes out, there are references on the news shows to an article in the new issue about some disease or some form of treatment before the magazine has even reached the physicians' mailboxes. It makes a difference in how medicine is practiced because the doctor has to be up on so many things and has to have an answer for questions about them. Sometimes, patients without a medical background will misinterpret things that they see in various periodicals or on television. While I don't know much about the Internet, I understand there is even more information on the Internet telling people where to go and what to do for all sorts of things. I predict that this is going to make the practice of medicine considerably more challenging than it is now.

HOSPITAL STAYS

The fact that patients are not staying in the hospital more than two or three days, sometimes after fairly extensive surgery—compared to the prior week or ten days—has the potential for quite a few side effects. One that impresses me is that the doctors don't have the chance to really get to know the patients. Back when we kept the patients with major operations in the hospital for a week, sometimes as long as ten days, calling on them—making rounds—once or twice a day, it not only helped to be sure they were doing all right, but also allowed us to get to know them well.

Many surgical patients have only been seen once or twice in the office. They were referred by somebody else, and the surgeon really doesn't have an idea what the patient is like emotionally. That comes to light when they are in the hospital, and although sometimes that can't be helped, a longer stay would allow the physician to better explore her needs. I think especially of breast cancer patients after a mastectomy. I would try to explain to a patient before the surgery about the disease, but at that time, she would be upset and wouldn't always pay attention to what was actually said. Immediately after that, she has had a biopsy, and the biopsy is positive, and the mastectomy is scheduled. She wakes up with her breast gone and has all the fears of and problems with what might be called "bodily mutilation."

If that patient were to go home two days after that, there wouldn't be a chance to talk to her about it and help her get over the immediate shock. On the other hand if she were in the hospital for five or six days, as she was when I was doing these operations, there would be an opportunity to see what her reaction is and help her with it and even get other help if necessary.

I know, on some occasions, I have had a cancer survivor who had a mastectomy come in to see my postoperative patient, and shown her that they could play tennis afterward—that it is not the end of the world. But with this business of getting them right out of the hospital, all of that is gone by the board. There is just no time to identify the issues or observe evolving medical complications in order to do anything about them.

One thing that I don't understand about short stays in the hospital is the system that is now in effect for patients coming in for operations. We used to have a patient come in the afternoon before—say at three o'clock. During that day, they got the lab work and the chest x-ray and the

EKG and any other preoperative tests. Then the doctor was able to see them on evening rounds, talk to them about last details and answer any of their questions or those of their family about the surgery. Then they were given a sedative, had a good night's sleep and woke up in the morning somewhat rested.

Now, the patient might be sent to the hospital two or three days before the surgery, unless it is an emergency. They have the lab work done as an outpatient, and the anesthetist sees them. It takes several hours out of that day for them. Then they go home without seeing their regular doctor.

On the day of the operation, they have to be in the hospital early in the morning for preparations. This means, in many cases—especially if they have come from any distance at all—that they are getting up before five o'clock in the morning to come into the hospital. Then they have the preps, are finally ready for surgery at eight or nine o' clock and are exhausted by the time it starts. Certainly, it is hard for the family, getting up that early, having to go into the hospital and then waiting. And it could have an effect on healing. However, this is the way it is done now.

TECHNOLOGY

Telemedicine has also brought changes. One or two experimental things are being done now. For instance, there is a project with Boston medical centers that has been going for several years now—a very complicated hook-up with Logan Airport. If a patient deplanes with symptoms of coronary disease or heart disease or heart failure, someone can put a stethoscope on his chest at the airport and a cardiologist at Massachusetts General can listen to the heart, watch the electrocardiogram and give advice on emergency treatment before the patient gets to the hospital.

This is not a new concept. For years telemedicine has assisted isolated towns all over the country where a hook-up can be made. A family practitioner of such a community can get a specialist of some type on hook-up with him or her and get advice on what to do. While I was in medical school, one of my professors was Dr. Elliott P. Joslin, the world-renowned authority on diabetes and founder of the Joslin Diabetes Clinic in Boston in 1898. In the mid-to-late '30s, he treated a seaman with diabetic coma over the wireless for two or three days until the ship could get into port.

There have been instances of individuals getting sick on private yachts and being helped through remote communication. Near the Galapagos Islands, a man and his wife were in a sailboat, and the man got symptoms that the wife thought she recognized as acute appendicitis. There were no ships with doctors in the area. Finally, she was patched through on her radio to San Diego, California, and the doctors there told her what to do. She followed the instructions to pack him in ice and eliminate anything by mouth. The man kept getting worse as she was trying to make port—I believe in Panama. Finally, they dispatched a destroyer with a doctor on it. The man had surgery on the destroyer and survived. There was a book written about it. This was about 50 years ago.

A significant expense of modern office practice is the technical equipment necessary. Neurologists want to have a very expensive MRI machine or CAT scanner or both. In other offices, it may be laser equipment needed for certain procedures. Not only is it expensive, but when the intervention is later replaced by some other procedure, it requires a completely different instrument.

Sometimes equipment lasts for only about three years before it is outdated, and this makes for a very expensive office.

When I first started practice in the early 1950s, there was a formula that I could use to easily figure what I was making. Most practices figured that 20% of charges could not be collected, 30% of the charges would go for overhead, and 50% of the charges would be profit. Now that is all different.

In some instances, a problem with medicine today is that some of the prices for interventions are outlandish—very high and not justified—although the interventions for which patients are charged don't require a great deal of skill or thought or care. Unfortunately, the overhead for running an office has gone up so much, the expenses have to be covered somehow.

Some technological advances also bring major problems with them—some of them are ethical issues. Fertility drugs are an example. The problem is that fertility drugs can lead to a large number of fetuses conceived at once; anything over triplets raises tremendously the risk of difficulties—not only for the mother, but for the fetuses. Single pregnancies are best statistically for both the baby and the mother. Twins are somewhat higher risk and triplets have significant jeopardy. After that, the risk goes up very steeply.

With high-order multiple births, a fair number of babies just don't live because of prematurity, but with the great increase in knowledge in the area of neonatal treatments, very small babies are being saved now which were not for most of the years of my obstetrical practice. However, many of these babies are badly damaged. They may have severe mental retardation or cerebral palsy or other severe neurological deficits, and if they live, that can be a tremendous burden on the families. The financial burden falls not only on the family, but on society in general.

There are ways of handling fertility drugs that obviate some of this. Ultrasound studies will tell whether or not the mother is going to ovulate and how many eggs she is going to ovulate. If there are quite a few—four, five, six, eight eggs—the physician can just call things off and wait another month before having the patient try to get pregnant. The next time, she could be given a different dose of the fertility drug, and if she ovulates three or fewer eggs, she could go ahead and try to get pregnant. There is a method—it was after my time and I don't know the technique of it—whereby the fertility specialist can destroy several of the fertilized eggs down to a number where two or three should develop. Of course, it is up to the parents in consultation with the physician, to decide whether or not they want to do this. It raises tremendous ethical questions that have to be settled. Fertilization in vitro has less risk of high-order multiple births. Because the sperm and egg are united outside the womb, the specialist knows how many ova have been fertilized and has control over how many are introduced into the uterus. This is usually more than one because some of the fertilized ova might not take.

MEDICAL ETHICS

The question of whether our ethics as human beings have kept up with technological developments is being debated every day. Most hospitals now have ethics committees which pass on whether research or various treatments should be done in a certain field—how one decides when to turn off the resuscitating machines and other matters of moral philosophy.

I think we've improved the response to the issue of keeping the life-support machines going, such as through living wills. I believe care should always be taken to analyze whether there is any hope for improvement before a final decision is made. A major problem nowadays would be when to stop tube feeding. There have been several lengthy court cases on that issue. I have already addressed the complexity of the ethics of reproductive technology.

I think that, generally, the ethics of medicine are good. Like everything else in medicine and business, certain individuals believe certain things. Who is to say who is right and who is wrong? Of course, there are some challenges with varying faiths and religious beliefs.

One of the areas of Ob/Gyn that has undergone significant change in the past 50 years is that of treating infertility. This field of medicine has become a subject of increasing controversy. For instance, the procedure that produces so-called test-tube babies has received a good bit of ethical scrutiny. An egg is removed from the mother, fertilized by sperm outside her body and replaced in the uterus, leading to a full-term baby. I personally do not see any reason for objecting to it. If there is a woman who cannot have a baby but who has perfectly good eggs and her husband has normal sperm, and if it is possible to get the egg and sperm together outside the mother and then implant it in her uterus so that she is able to have a normal baby, there is merit in the great happiness it brings for the couple.

I believe that some find objection to the procedures on religious as well as ethical bases. If sperm from other than the husband were used, some might have a problem with that, although it seems to me that is a private matter for the donor and the mother and the husband . . . if there is a husband.

The business of freezing sperm seems to be a perfectly acceptable situation. If it's not the husband's sperm that is used, it's no different from artificial insemination used in cases of married couples where the husband did not have a good sperm count. This was a procedure we learned when I was in medical school. We did find that there could be considerable trouble in a case where a husband's brother's sperm was used, so selected to keep the genes those of the family. We found that if the mother knew the source of the sperm, there could be a transference of affection to the genetic father of the baby. That might cause all sorts of emotional problems in the family. It was decided long ago that in artificial insemination, the mother should not have any idea of the identity of the donor.

I question whether this procedure should be used on single girls just so they can have a baby if they want one. The fact that single women sometimes get sperm from a sperm bank and are inseminated seems to me to pose some ethical questions. I don't know if there is a definite answer as to what is right or wrong in this situation. I believe the main consideration should be whether this single mother can raise the child well. She may have plenty of money but might not be able to provide a family environment for the child—absent a father's influence. I would think that probably there would be some cases where it was advisable. One of the considerations might be the reason that the woman is single. A woman who has had a husband who died young might be an example in support of the procedure. I couldn't give a definite answer as to whether it would be as good a thing or not. I've seen so many people, some of them married, who simply have to have a baby because other people have them and it's expected of them, but they are just not emotionally capable of taking care of the child.

The solution of using surrogate mothers became popular in recent years. A woman is artificially inseminated with the sperm of the man of the infertile couple. The recipient substitutes for his wife who is unable to carry a baby. After the baby is delivered, it is then adopted back by the married couple so that at least the child has genes from both. I don't know that there is anything wrong with this except the possibility that the mother who has the child—the birth mother—might eventually want the baby back, especially if she knows who the parents are and where the child is. It seems to me that there is a considerable possibility that later she could attempt to adopt or get possession of the child, particularly if the child becomes some person of renown. I think these emotionally-laden situations could come up and even be dangerous. But on the other hand, the availability of a surrogate mother does give a barren couple the chance to have children, raise them and have the happiness that comes from that experience. One has to balance the negative with the positive, and I don't know that there is a clear answer in each case.

I guess I am a little more practical than some of my colleagues. I can't, for the life of me, see what is wrong with in-vitro fertilization for a couple who can't have babies. If the wife has had her tubes removed, but there are ovaries, they are functioning well and her uterus is healthy, why shouldn't the couple be allowed to have their own genetic children—by uniting the sperm and egg in the laboratory and then placing the conceptus in the womb? Certain faiths are dead-set against it. That doesn't make sense to me.

My own personal ethics in matters that arise in medicine tend to lean toward what the patient wants. Certainly, I would not put a family through having to cope for years with a child who just had no mentality at all and who had severe physical defects along with it. I have seen too many of these families break apart over such a problem. I would not kill such a baby, but I would not work hard to resuscitate the infant, and I would not advocate that a lot of things be done in the nursery to keep the child alive.

The question of abortion is a very difficult thing. I certainly don't support using abortion as birth control. People who are able to use birth control shouldn't rely on abortion. I've seen a great many babies born before we could do abortions legally whose mothers, when they found out they were pregnant, were very upset and wanted an illegal abortion, but by the time the baby moved or at least by the time the baby came, they wanted the child very badly. So I think great care has to be taken there. But suppose it is a fifteen-year-old girl in high school whose family does not have any resources. That, I think, is a whole different story.

At the other end of life, I've had experience with some people who have very severe Alzheimer's disease. They finally are placed in a nursing home where they lie like a log with no response to anybody or anything—absolutely zero quality of life. I certainly don't believe in tube feeding or in giving them antibiotics to keep them alive. I wouldn't want it for myself, and I wouldn't push it on anybody else. I guess my ethics, in many ways, boil down to doing what the family wants or the patient wants after everything is reviewed with consultation and careful discussion.

CHANGING IDEAS

I never got very involved with political issues such as the Vietnam War. For one thing, the war came at a time when I was the busiest. I was overwhelmed with the practice, working literally day and night. I had the feeling then, which

I now know was wrong, that the government should know what it was doing. If they felt it was necessary, then I went along, and I didn't question the motives of the government as I would now. That was how I was brought up—people in Washington knew what they were doing and you supported them. That was how we felt in WWII. We had ample evidence of what we were fighting for and against—the enemies were Hitler and Stalin and their ways.

In fact, during the Vietnam War years, I was against the student marches. I couldn't understand why the universities acted the way they did when students rebelled, went into the president's office and tore up records. I thought those people should have been arrested, certainly thrown out of the university and not given any sounding board. I still believe that's not the way to settle things.

There was an incident at Harvard in which I couldn't understand why Harvard Medical School acted as it did. This didn't have anything to do with the Vietnam War. The medical school is in Boston, not in Cambridge. Harvard had bought up large residential areas around the school. The area was composed mostly of townhouses. The school had kept it for some years, renting those places. They wanted to control the area for when they had to expand. The time for expansion came. I don't know exactly when this was, probably in the 1970s. They gave the people who were renting those facilities three years before they would have to get out; then they planned to demolish the housing. The medical students—a large portion of them—rebelled and went on strike on the basis that these were people's homes, and the university had no right to tell them they had to leave their homes—in spite of three years' notice.

I'm sure that in my day, for a lot less than that, the school would have said, "Well, you go on your way, student. We have a lot of other people who want to come to Harvard Medical School." I couldn't understand how the school tolerated that behavior and gave it any credence at all. I still can't. When I was in medical school—and my classmates were the same way—we were so glad to be there, to be chosen over four or five thousand people. Whatever the faculty said was okay with us, and we were not going to challenge it. Another such incident involved classes on Saturday morning. We had been required to attend each week until 1:00 p.m. Some years later, when students everywhere around the country began telling people what they would and wouldn't do, on the very first day of classes in September, the first-year class announced to the faculty that they were not going to attend any Saturday classes. Students decided Saturday classes were a thing of the past. I can't imagine what would have happened if we had done that. None of us would have ever considered that in my student days.

MISSION WORK

In 1973 Betty went with me to Haiti. She had been an operating room nurse. At Haiti she worked in the medical supply area. Half the time the lights would go out in the middle of surgery, requiring completion of the operation with an assistant holding flashlights. My slogan was, "If you didn't do it, who would?" Some people would walk for two days to get to the hospital, like one woman who previously had a traumatic delivery. Someone had to use forceps, and she had seven holes in her bladder. Repairing that was a challenge.

I worked in Haiti at an outpatient clinic at the hospital. A well-trained, native registered nurse would come in and work with the patients until I finished operating. One day he came to the operating room for me. I finished surgery and followed him back to the clinic. There were only curtains around each examining table. They seldom got pulled. This time, the curtains were drawn around one bed even though there weren't any other people there. The Haitian patient was as beautiful a woman as I had ever seen. Given what little I knew about female attire, I thought her clothing had to be from Paris. I inquired about her problem. She said a native doctor in the city had said she had an ovarian tumor that had to come out right away. I glanced out a window at that moment and saw a huge black limousine with a chauffeur. I examined her. She had very normal pelvic anatomy. I explained my findings and told her she didn't need surgery. She thanked me very graciously, got up and left. I learned she was a wife or friend or relative of some high official. After she left, my RN assistant said, "Doctor, do you know what you've done?"

"No. I didn't find anything wrong."

"The MD down in the city will be lucky if he has not been shot by nightfall."

The month I spent in Haiti, operating in the little mission hospital with very poor facilities, permanently changed my idea of disadvantaged people around the world. Until then, I had not been very sympathetic with a lot of the cultures I knew anything about because I felt the people were not trying to help themselves. For instance, I heard a lot about the starving people in India, and yet they wouldn't kill cattle for food because they were sacred. I would take the attitude, Why send money over there to them? Let them do what they can for themselves first—then help them after that if they need it.

But after I had been to Haiti and had seen the abject poverty there and the difficulties with the dictatorial regime of Baby Doc, and after I had been close to the people, seeing the state they were in, I realized that they could not help themselves. They couldn't get an education. They couldn't move from one strata of society to the next. They just had to use all of their energy to survive.

I remember delivering a set of premature twins there that weighed about two-and-a-half or three pounds. We worked hard to save them. But then the realization came over me that after they left the hospital, they probably wouldn't live more than two or three days because there was no way anybody could take care of them. There were no formulas, and the mother probably couldn't nurse both of them. Those types of things were hard to come to grips with emotionally and intellectually.

This made an impact on me as far as my charitable giving went. It changed my attitude toward mission work around the world. I was not a person who was going to try and go back down there and overthrow the government or anything like that. I guess I work more by example than anything else.

It was the same way here in Asheville. When I found out that there wasn't any prenatal clinic when I first arrived in 1947, I went ahead and started one and did the best I could with it. I wasn't one to go out and start a campaign to have the hospitals integrated. I just tried to work by example and give the best care I could to the people—whether they could pay or not.

VALUES

As I reflect on my life, I have remembered several things that have helped to shape my personality. I was brought up in a family that had a pretty sound value system. I remember how I was taught by example.

During the days when I was in school, there were tramps going through the country. They would rap on the back door and ask my mother for something to eat. She would always give them quite a meal. My brother, who had gone to college before I did, came back one time on vacation and a tramp came in. Mother fussed around getting him nice food. My brother knew everything that could be known at that age. In those days, we had a great many people who today would be classified as homeless. They went through the country and would stop at a house and try to get a meal. They often would then get back on an empty freight car and travel quite a ways. After the tramp was gone, my brother said, "She shouldn't be doing that. That man will tell all of his acquaintances on the road that you were an easy touch; you will have a lot people coming by wanting meals. So many of them don't deserve it."

Mother overheard his remarks. She said, "I'd rather help nine undeserving than have one deserving go hungry."

This made an impression on me. I've always tried to apply that to whatever decisions I face regarding doing things for people. I think it had something to do with my never turning anyone away from the office, no matter what their situation was. I have tried to live that philosophy along the way in other aspects of life also.

As long as I can remember, I understood that honesty was the thing to do and that serving others was a laudable practice. I don't think I ever put money high up on the list. I did want enough money to feel secure in retirement. I saw my parents struggle through the Depression and end up with barely enough money to live comfortably in their retirement. That made me determined not to earn a lot of money and then just waste it.

"Anger destroys the vessel that contains it." This was said by one of the people I've been friends with a long time, a counselor. I have thought about it over and over again. I know a great many people whose lives are destroyed by hanging onto an anger toward somebody else. It may break up a family because of anger toward a family member that cannot be resolved. I've seen that to be true so often, I try not to get angry at people, and, if it flashes up, I try not to let it stay. I think anger is a very poor thing to have in one's repertoire.

I learned that there is value in laying a sound foundation and then building on it. I remember when I entered medical school, the great Dr. Horax granted me an interview. I didn't realize what a great man he was at the time. I wasn't very much in awe of him. We had a pleasant hour, which I am sure he carved out of a very busy schedule. Near the end of the interview, he asked, "Is there anything I could do to help you?"

I said, "It would be interesting if I could come and see you operate sometime."

His reply was, "No, that is not anything you need to do. You need to concentrate on getting as good a basic medical education as you can. The operating can come later. For now, don't waste your time coming to see me operate. Work hard to establish the best foundation that you can."

I always remembered that, and in the years that followed, I told medical students that same thing. Never mind the fancy things, go for the basics. I always wanted to keep getting better, and so I suppose I had a fear of mistakes. I certainly didn't want to make any dumb mistakes. I wanted to be the very best I could be.

ALTRUISM

Most of us had this idea many years ago that we went into medicine to help the patient, and many still do, but more and more, the emphasis on the financial aspects and time off is taking over and ruling how medicine is practiced. The financial aspects of medicine have to take more of a back seat. The idea of service has to come into play more—not only with the doctors but with the paramedical staff. The whole thing has to evolve into a system where the service presented is paramount and not the amount of money made. All of this takes a complete turnaround from the way things are at the moment.

10

FAMILY

I expect I see part of myself in my children and grandchildren. I don't know of any specific traits, but all three of my daughters are very hard working and do the best they can to succeed in whatever they do. It is very good for us to see the grandchildren succeed in school or sports. I enjoy watching them compete at basketball or ride in horse shows. I enjoyed the experience in New York when two of my daughters rode in Madison Square Garden in the national championship and when I went to other cities where they were riding. Later—one generation later—I watched the two granddaughters, at different times, repeat the Madison Square Garden experience at the annual national horse show, qualifying for the McClay championship events. I remember with pride going to Washington to see some basketball games that they were playing in. All of this is very pleasing and helps with being retired—approaching the end of life.

At this stage of my life in retirement, I have time to think about some things. One of those things is how much

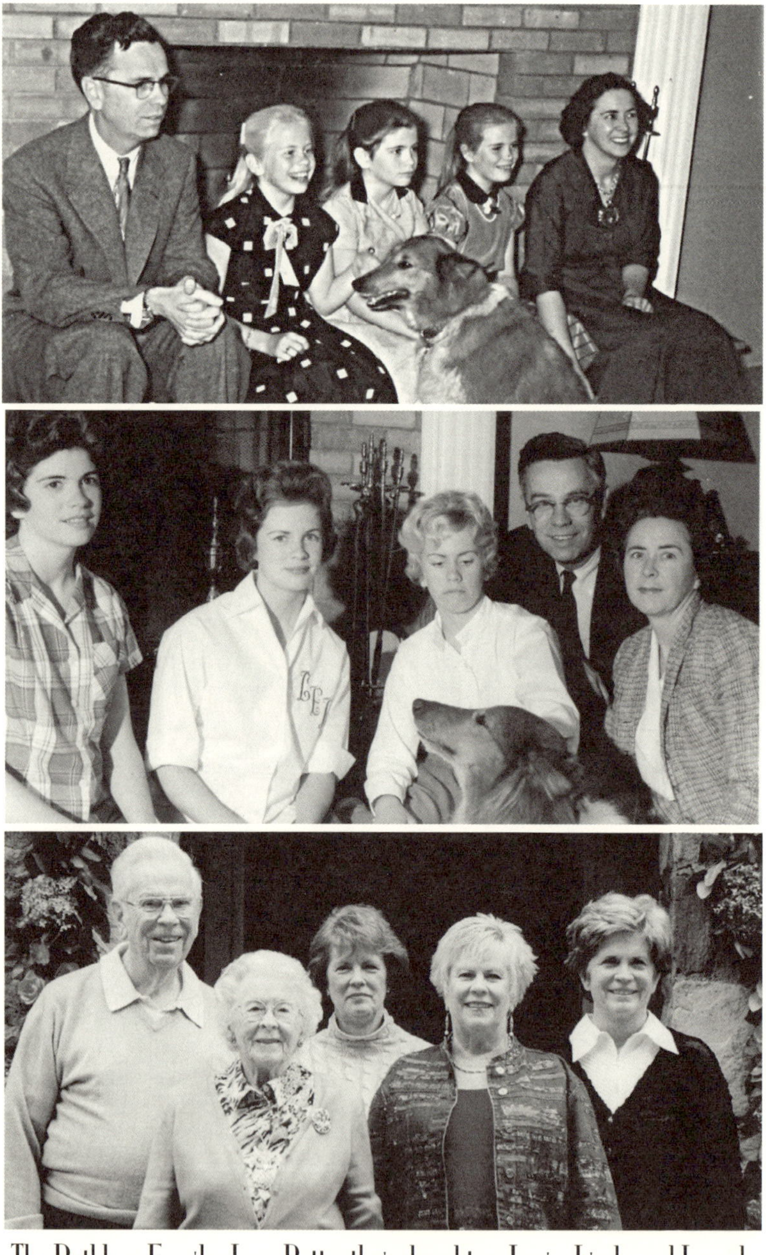

The Rathbun Family: Lew, Betty, their daughters Lexie, Linda and Laurel, and Sheba, the collie

my children and grandchildren mean to me. I look at some of my friends who are essentially the age of my wife and me and who are without children and wonder how they get along—what their interests are. It is so rewarding to see your children do well, to have them call and visit and to follow the course of the grandchildren. I have four granddaughters and one grandson.

We have had some special situations with the grandchildren. We have a granddaughter with Down syndrome. We also have a granddaughter who had a very serious head injury in which a large portion of her frontal lobes was destroyed. She has had considerable difficulty since that time. She is quite smart. Her writing abilities are wonderful. Both girls are so loving to me.

I expect I see part of myself in my children and grandchildren. I don't know of any specific traits, but all three of my daughters are very hard working and do the best they can to succeed in whatever they do. It is very good for us to see the grandchildren succeed in school or sports. I enjoy watching them compete at basketball or ride in horse shows. I enjoyed the experience of going to New York when two of my daughters rode in Madison Square Garden in the national championship and went to other cities where they were riding. I later—one generation later—watched the two granddaughters, at different times, repeat the Madison Square Garden experience at the annual national horse show, qualifying for the McClay championship events.

I remember with pride going to Washington to see some high school basketball games that they played in. My grandson keeps me up to date on all the professional football leagues. All of this is very satisfying and helps with being retired—approaching the end of your life.

With all the confusion there is now and the talk about how much parents have to do with whether children succeed or not, it is very comforting to see my children as quite successful people. It makes me think maybe I didn't do such a bad job after all. I think we have been blessed with our children.

It is also a great pleasure to me, barring some financial disaster, that I will be able to help them some by leaving them some money. So, as they grow older, they will be comfortable and secure in their old age. One of the goals I have had throughout my life—having lived through the depression—has been to want to have good security in my old age. I always said I wasn't going to squander money that I made. I worked hard to make it and saw no reason to lose it if I could possibly help it. By the same token, I felt that it was okay to spend it and be comfortable with it. One doesn't have to be miserly.

As I read biographies and realize how much time some parents—especially fathers—have spent with their children, I wonder quite a bit if I spent enough time with my girls. Right now, I am reading a biography of Theodore "Teddy" Roosevelt. Teddy's father, in spite of being a successful businessman, spent a tremendous amount of time with him doing things together. Because of my busy practice, I sometimes felt that I didn't spend as much time with the girls . . . or know them as well at that time of life as I should have.

CHILDREN

Lexie, my eldest, was born when I was over in the Pacific. She was about seven or eight months old when I got back after our ship was hit, and then I still had about a year in the Navy spent at the Naval Air Station in Atlanta. Betty and the baby came down there. The place I found for them to stay was not ideal, but it was the best I could find in all of Atlanta. That year I was on duty at the Naval Air Station taking care of dependents. The work wasn't all that rigorous so I was able to get home and enjoy the family—enjoy seeing Lexie take her first steps. When I got out of the Navy, I went to the clinic in Rockford, Illinois, and I worked very hard to try and build a practice. Even though I tried to stay on call all the time, it wasn't arduous and didn't take me away from the family too much. Betty got pregnant with Linda while I was in the Navy and delivered just before I got out, so when we went out there to Rockford, we had two, and I was able to spend time with them.

I never was terribly enthusiastic about young babies until they got old enough to develop some personality. Until then, they were just something to be taken care of. When they began to get personality, I was interested in their development and tried to spend some time with them. After a year in Rockford, it was obvious to me that I didn't want to stay in the clinic out there. I came to Asheville to provide Ob/Gyn services in a multispecialty practice. Ultimately, when I went out on my own after three years, I began to spend a great deal more time with my practice. It grew rapidly. I had always considered that practicing medicine was my main job in life and that it was Betty's job to take care of the family. So I didn't spend a lot of time with the children at that stage. Laurel was born shortly after we got to Asheville. We could afford household help. We lived right near the hospital so I was home nights, unless a patient was in labor.

It may seem ironic that although my work was delivering babies, when my children were babies, it was not as interesting to be involved. I don't personally look at it as an irony. The process of getting a woman through pregnancy and seeing her through to a successful delivery was a challenge and was something to be accomplished. After that, it was up to the pediatrician to take care of the baby.

I'm talking about babies up to three or four months. To me, they don't have much in the way of personality in that early time. I couldn't get down to their level. I wouldn't know how to be a pediatrician and spend all day with an office full of babies and worried mothers. Of course, it was a long time ago, and I may not remember what my emotions were.

I was interested in the well-being of my children—very interested in that. If they got sick, I was intent on seeing they had the best of everything.

I can't remember too much of my philosophy about child rearing, but I know that it is very important for children to have a father and a mother. Betty never worked after the babies started coming. I was there with them and reading to them, and I think that is tremendously important. The stability of the home is critical. I doubt very much that daycare centers, with two people in the family working, are a good way to bring up children, but I do recognize it is often necessary these days.

Family activities changed as the girls got older. When they were fairly small, we would go on picnics or to the circus. After they got a little bigger, I tried to do athletic things with them. We played badminton in the back yard, started going on picnics up in the mountains and went swimming at the country club.

I would have liked to have had some boys, but as I think on it now, I don't know how to raise boys. Once you have a couple of girls, it is pretty nice to have the third one as a girl. One gets into a path on how to bring up children of one gender. I think it might be difficult to switch to another one midstream.

My children influenced my life, my views, and my sense of who I am. I was always proud of them. I was proud of their achievements in school. They were all good students. Lexie was an especially accomplished musician, a role she gave up when she discovered boys and the glamour of long fingernails. We were told by a pianist that she could go as far as she wanted in that field. But there was no fire in her to do it, although she did seem to enjoy it. She went on to be sought-after for community boards and projects. Linda turned out to be one of the best equestrians in the country during high school and the years that followed. She was always one to work at everything she did. Laurel was also a good student. She spent more time reading. She loves animals. She has written two very successful books on the subject of grieving the loss of a pet.

I tried to set a good example, especially regarding the work ethic. I tried to give them an idea of values.

The girls didn't give us trouble with adolescence. They all went to Country Day School. It was sheltered. Then we had a learning experience with Lexie when she was going into the seventh grade. We were talked into transferring her to the public junior high school by other parents who said she would benefit from the diversity. It wasn't very long before we began to hear that "only nerds went to college." We tried to combat that attitude. It was obvious that the school wasn't challenging her to work up to her potential. I went over to talk to her teacher one day by appointment and found a woman who had children of her own. She was getting through teaching about 3:30 in the afternoon and having to go home and do all her own housework and take care of her own children. She seemed just too worn out to do much in the way of working with the children in her class. After a year of that, we sent Lexie to St. Genevieve's. She finished high school there. The school had a good record. I remember at one of the dances at St. Genevieve's, I was signed up as a chaperone. My job was to spend the evening in the boy's restroom to see that they didn't have liquor in flasks and drink it in there.

The three children are so different. There is some of me in each. I see the work ethic both in Lexie and Linda, and to a different degree in Laurel. Laurel has been successful, but it took her awhile to find where she was. Now she works very hard at her occupation and is doing a very good job. Linda has some of the same interests as mine. But none of the girls wanted to be a doctor. We never tried to push them into one field or another; we let them make their own paths. Lexie went to college mainly for the social aspects. She did well, but she didn't take any higher math or anything like that. Immediately after graduation, she became an airline flight attendant because she liked being with people. She liked traveling, and she liked the days off. She would work three to four days and then had three to four days off. She did that for 23 years. She didn't seek intellectual challenges. She was always good company, but she always thought that we were pretty much sticks in the mud.

Linda was a student from the word go. She was valedictorian of her class at Country Day. She graduated cum laude from Vassar and was vice-president of her senior class, then graduated from Harvard Business School cum laude.

She was a mathematics major and a good student. I was very proud of her. They had a Father's Weekend for the sophomore class at Vassar, and I went up there. We had a wonderful experience, just the two of us. We went to a dance; there I was dancing with this good-looking young girl. We went to some classes. I look back on that as a very happy and exciting time.

Laurel was also valedictorian of her class and then went to Cornell. She was a shy type of person. She didn't seem to make friends easily. She loved Cornell for about a year and a half. After not being accepted by a desired sorority, she didn't enjoy the rest of her college time anywhere near as much as she did the first part. I didn't realize that at the time, or I would have tried to talk to her and correct it.

It was not easy juggling family and obstetrics. I just plain went when I got a call to come to the hospital . I felt like that was what I was there for. That's what people hired me for. I remember one Christmas Day, when I delivered three babies, that it didn't interfere with either our tree or Christmas dinner. The babies just came at the right time. I remember Christmases with the family as fun times.

I remember one Christmas when the girls were as excited as the dickens on Christmas Eve. We finally got them to bed. We brought the presents out, set them around the tree and then turned in ourselves. There were a couple of things, like Lexie's first bicycle and a few dolls that weren't wrapped. At 12:30, I got a call and had to go to the hospital. In spite of being as quiet as I could be, they all woke up and went tearing out. There was the tree with all the wrapped presents and the bicycle and the dolls. We had another job getting them back to bed. We usually were up by 5:30 or 6:00 a.m. on Christmas day. I have some pictures of those early Christmases. The pictures show us opening presents and when the camera was pointed toward the window, they show it was black as pitch outside. They understood what my job was.

If I could go back and do anything differently, I would spend more time with the kids, or try to, when they were smaller—two, three or four years old. I spent a lot of time with them though, as much as I possibly could.

When they got into horses, I would haul the horses around and go to all the shows. I did my very best. In fact, one of the major points of family life for a long time was the girls' interest in horses. It gave me a chance to get closer to them and have activities with them. It started with Linda, the middle girl, when she was about five. She decided in the fall that Santa Claus was going to give her a horse for Christmas.

We kept saying that we didn't have any place to keep a horse. But she kept insisting that Santa was going to bring her a horse. So we inquired around and found a very small bridle and saddle club out in the Biltmore area where there were two ladies who, just as a hobby, were teaching young children to ride. There was a very small charge involved. We bought a certificate for ten lessons and gave it to her at Christmas time instead of giving her a horse. She was very enthusiastic about the lessons, and about the time she had finished ten, the other two girls wanted lessons, so they all took up horseback riding. They had little ponies that just trotted and trotted and trotted. The girls couldn't fall off, because the little horses' necks were so wide.

Then they had a couple of little shows, and Linda got her first blue ribbon as a beginner in one of them. Next, Laurel got a ribbon. So we kept this up, progressing into horses that were a little more difficult to ride. Then came the inevitable: I had to buy a horse. I didn't know a thing about buying a horse, but we found a fellow out in the country who had one. I remember I paid him $50. (Linda is now paying $350,000 for a horse.)

All three took turns riding that first horse. He was a good solid old fellow. Tryon, North Carolina, 36 miles south of Asheville, is a real horsey place with large estates, stables and fox hunting. So we progressed to going down to Tryon for lessons with a professional, who was an excellent teacher. Then I had to buy better horses. The girls became junior members of the Tryon Hunt and began going to some of the bigger shows around.

Then I had to buy a horse trailer and put a hitch on the car. Lexie, at about twelve- or thirteen-years old, lost interest. Although she didn't continue, the other two did. They started winning at shows in nearby towns.

Linda got to be a very good rider. Finally, when she was in high school, I bought her a young horse—four-and-a half years old—from one of the stables in Tryon. She continued training him, and he turned out to be a great horse. Unfortunately, he got very severe ankle problems, and we finally had to put him down when Linda was a sophomore in college. Needless to say, that was a great emotional blow for her.

Laurel also did well. One year in high school, both girls qualified for the national over fences junior championship at Madison Square Garden. I took them up there. Unfortunately, it was just frightfully expensive to get their horses up there, so I borrowed two horses. Their trainer knew horses inside and out, and he was up there at Madison Square Garden himself. He let Linda ride one of his and leased another horse from out on Long Island for Laurel. The latter one turned out to be a terrible choice. The horse was so confused in Madison Square Garden that he wouldn't do anything. Laurel tried her best. Finally, the horse crashed into a jump, and she and the horse went down.

I had a good time with the girls doing this and getting closer to them all the time. Linda has kept up her interest in horses, and now her two girls, my grandchildren, are getting to the top of the national ladder. They ride jumpers and hunters, and they go to the really big shows all over the country—from down in Florida to up in New England. That is a very costly affair. Fortunately, Linda and her husband have the money to carry it on. There is an area around Warrenton where they ride, and I go and see them when I am up that way. In fact, the same trainer, Arthur Reynolds, who worked in Tryon, had moved to the area—part of Virginia's well known horse country. He was still a superb teacher, and he was still saying his signature line, "You never be no better than your basics." He gave the grandchildren some early lessons. When I was up there, which wasn't often, I would go out and see him teaching my grandchildren, and it would take me back to the time he was teaching my daughters.

However, I did the best I could once they got into horses at age seven or eight—trailering horses around to horse shows, taking time off to do that. I was very proud of them for how well they did at the national championship event. I perhaps could have spent more money and had better horses, but I was also committed to the business of trying to save for their future.

I think my love has grown deeper and my anxiety has seemed to lessen as my daughters have grown older. Our relationships grew rapidly after they reached an age for us to talk to each other. That made it more satisfying.

I never had a lot of chance to play with my grandchildren. We enjoyed Christmas—playing with the toys. It was after they got to be active, doing things like children's soccer, and began to get into the horses, that I shared more time with them. I took pride in their accomplishments in school. I used to try to show them this by writing them encouraging letters when we heard they had gotten all A's or succeeded at something. I still do that with the basketball and the horses, when they've had a particularly outstanding show in top competition. I write them a letter to put their ego up and try to help their self-esteem.

GRANDCHILDREN

Education is so different with the grandchildren from the way it was with our children. What I hear now about the teaching of geography, for instance, amazes me. In our days we knew the Ganges River started in India and emptied into the Indian Ocean, and the Amazon started up in the Andes and ended in the Atlantic Ocean. We memorized all of that—the capital of Brazil is Brasilia, the five oceans are Atlantic, Pacific, Indian . . .

When something comes up, now for instance, in the Middle East, about Baghdad and the Euphrates River and the war over there, the youth today have no idea where the Euphrates River is. We learned it by rote. I don't know that it did us a great deal of good to learn it like that. It was the same way I felt about organic chemistry in medical school. We needed to know the theories of organic chemistry, but we didn't have to spend two hours on how to do a blood sugar analysis in the lab, because most of us were never going to be doing that procedure. If we were, we could learn it then. I always thought that chemistry labs in medical school were really a waste of time. Nowadays, I don't think students do much of that.

There are times when not enough is learned. If I were giving my grandchildren advice, I think it would be, whatever you study, do it well. Learn a broad base. When I went to college, we studied Romance languages, history and English literature. As a freshman, you had to take everything—including freshman math. Then, in the second year, the class choices became more flexible. I had a good foundation. If somebody talks about Chaucer, I know what they are talking about. I'm not an authority on it, but at least I know. But I wouldn't have known if I had just taken the courses I needed to get into medical school.

The same thing is true about medical school. Several years ago, there was a boy I knew whose father died and left me, not to watch over him, but to show an interest in him. The boy wanted to go to medical school, and I gave him some advice at the time. When he was about to begin his fourth year, he wrote me and said that he could spend three months in Australia doing some dermatology over there. I wrote back and said he would be much better to stay in the USA and use that time to broaden his knowledge—broaden his base with intensive study in his own medical school. The time to go to Australia and study dermatology was when he was a resident—if he decided he wanted to do dermatology.

The idea is for a student to keep his or her knowledge base as broad as possible before specializing. I would tell my grandchild, "Get a broad, firm base in everything that you can. Keep your knowledge. It's going to come up. It might help you to know something about Shakespeare, for instance. If there's interest in a career in the computer industry, it might help first to get some background in engineering. You really need a broad base until you get to what you are going to do."

REFLECTIONS ON CHILDREARING

I don't think that there is very much, as far as bringing up children, that you can tell other people. Situations are so different and every person is so different. You just have to use your head, try to be logical and do what seems to be called for when facing each problem. I certainly wouldn't consider myself an authority on how to bring up wonderful children. I learned over the years not to try to press older children to do things that they are downright against such as a particular job or college or playing a sport just because I did—if they didn't want it.

I think that getting a divorce can be very deleterious to children, although, of course, you can say also—and I'm sure it's true—that living in a household with no love and with fighting all the time is also deleterious. I think a lot of children of divorced parents turn out to be very unstable. They are left with the thought, *One of them has left me, and what have I done that they wanted to leave me?* They may also have a fear, if they are younger, *Well, Daddy left me or Mommy left me; maybe the other one will leave me, too, and where will I be then?* I think it is mostly subconscious, but I'm sure it's there. I think that any couple with children should consider long and hard before they get a divorce.

Speaking of life in general, my advice would be to use your own head. Here's an example:

Years ago, I was still in high school when my brother came back and went into business with my father. He was eight years older than I was and lived at the house. He was single at the time, so we had plenty of opportunity to get very close together. I couldn't drive, and we would sometimes go on double dates. He would have a date, and I would have a date with one of my school friends—when I was 14 or 15. In those days, there might be a pavilion where there was a dance band scheduled, so we would go there to dance. I've forgotten some of the details, but we paid 25 cents a dance. We bought tickets and then went out on the dance floor. If you really liked the girl, that could be a special time.

We had some great conversations on those outings. I've never forgotten what my brother once said to me. "In deciding whether I ought to do something or not, I think to myself, *What would happen if everybody in the world did this? What would the world be like?*"

I picked up that habit. When I was asked to do something like a civic project or church work that I didn't really care about doing, I would ask myself, *Suppose nobody would do this. Then what would it be like?* If I felt I would like to have done whatever was proposed, but I didn't want to be the one to do it, I realized that if everybody took my attitude, then it wouldn't get done. Yet it should get done, so I would do it.

I think there is a fair amount of research showing that there are a great many people who have nothing to do with churches, but if they were to be asked, "Would you like to live in a town with no churches?" they would say, "Oh no, I wouldn't."

A lot of other things go the same way. I once asked a person whom I knew well to help me with a community-type job, and got the answer, "I don't have enough time to do the things I want to do in life, so I'm certainly not going to do the things I don't want to do." I felt like asking him what he thought the place would be like if everybody had that attitude.

EPILOGUE

I feel, as I look back, how lucky I was—how privileged—to grow up in a stable family without a lot of divorces and with a fairly religious background. My youth had few of the things that get so many young people today into so much trouble. I had a loving family—a family that sacrificed more than I knew at the time to put me through college and medical school. I feel extremely grateful to my mother and father for making it possible.

I have been able to get an excellent education in spite of the Depression. I feel very good about having gone to Hamilton, a small college where I could get to know the professors and my fellow classmates. It was another stable environment. We didn't have much money to spend. I think there were only three people on campus who had a car—quite different from today. It was during prohibition, so there was no liquor on campus. There was one Speakeasy we could go to, but no one had the money to do it.

The decision to go into the service was mine. I saw a lot of the negative side of war—the extremes of human hatred—but took great pride in defending my country.

I really think that by coming up at the exact time that I did, it shaped me to work hard and do the very best I could. I feel extremely grateful to my teachers in medical school. They were a fine group of men—tops in their fields. It was a privilege to work with them, especially in residency—to operate with them and see how they made diagnoses and decisions. I'm grateful for the patients who taught me a great deal about medicine. That career led to the fulfilling work with Life After Cancer.

And I treasure the opportunities to express myself through art in retirement.

Betty has done so much through the years to promote the life of our family, our girls and their families now. My words here fall short of expressing how much each of them mean to me. I feel that people who reach this stage of retirement and who have no children are missing so much by not having a family to communicate with and to share the young people's hopes and desires and their success and problems. It is one of the finest things in the late years.

So, all in all, I have had a wonderful life. I have had the privilege of fulfilling my early-life desire of becoming a doctor. The honors that have been bestowed on me mean a great deal to me. They are not what I was working toward. I was working to be the very best physician I could be and one who served people.

For me medicine has been a very satisfying life's work. I am certainly glad I went into it and hope that I did a good job. I feel that I did. I believe that I have been able to do a lot more good than harm in this life. This is one of the things that makes me very happy.

My medical school class celebrated its 60th reunion in June of 1999. A preponderance of surviving class members—which were not many—stated that they saw medicine now becoming a business. They almost unanimously agreed that this was deleterious to the practice of medicine as we had known it through the years and as we had practiced it—as we think it should be practiced.

PATHWAYS
LIFE AFTER CANCER

At the time of publication, Life After Cancer continues to help patients in Asheville, North Carolina, through the Cancer Center of Mission Hospital. The author is donating a portion of his royalties from the sale of this book to Life After Cancer.

– logo reprinted by permission

The Rathbun Center

a welcoming place to stay.

logo reprinted by permission

The House with a Heart
has served over 14,000 people.

I am deeply indebted to Adelaide Key, founder of The Rathbun Center. She saw the need for a place for people to stay—patients and their relatives from the outlying communities—who came in for services at Mission Hospital.

The Rathbun House graciously offered free rent to Life After Cancer for meeting purposes.

ABOUT THE AUTHOR

Dr. Lewis S. Rathbun made an early decision to become a physician. As a boy, he followed the rural family doctor on housecalls, practiced operating on a cat and studied with great interest the reactions of his relatives to ill health. He noted at quite a young age that emotions seemed to influence wellness and illness. He received his medical school education at Harvard, a two-year internship at Strong Memorial Hospital in Rochester, New York, and a three-year residency in the Obstetrics-Gynecology Department at Harvard. He served his country in battle in World War II, as a physician aboard a PT Tender.

One of the first Ob-Gyn specialists in Asheville, North Carolina, he demonstrated optimum qualities of a physician—thoroughness, dedication, altruism. He was committed to treating both mind and body of his patients and founded Life After Cancer in Asheville, North Carolina, a program with a mission to help people with cancer improve the quality of their lives by providing counseling, education and other resources that promote healing and may ultimately change the course of their disease.

The father of three grown daughters, Lexie, Linda and Laurel, Dr. Rathbun lives in Asheville, North Carolina, with his wife, Betty.